Biological Centrifugation

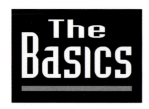

Series Advisors:

Rob Beynon UMIST, Manchester, UK
Chris Howe Department of Biochemistry, University of Cambridge, Cambridge, UK

Monoclonal Antibodies
PCR
Analyzing Chromosomes
Separating Cells
Biological Centrifugation

Forthcoming titles

Gene Mapping
Reconstructing Evolutionary Trees

Biological Centrifugation

John Graham

John Graham Research Consultancy, Wirral, Merseyside, UK

© BIOS Scientific Publishers Limited, 2001

First published 2001

A CIP catalogue record for this book is available from the British Library.

ISBN 1 85996 037 5

BIOS Scientific Publishers Ltd
9 Newtec Place, Magdalen Road, Oxford OX4 1RE, UK
Tel. +44 (0)1865 726286. Fax +44 (0)1865 246823
World Wide Web home page: http://www.bios.co.uk/

Distributed in the United States of America, its dependent territories, Canada, Mexico, Central and Sou America, and the Caribbean by Springer-Verlag New York Inc., 175 Fifth Avenue, New York, USA, t arrangement with BIOS Scientific Publishers, Ltd, 9 Newtec Place, Magdalen Road, Oxford OX4 1RE, U

Production Editor: Paul Barlass
Typeset by J&L Composition Ltd., N Yorks, UK
Printed by TJ International, Padstow, Cornwall, UK

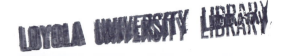

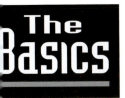

Contents

**List of manufacturers and technical
support sources**   2(

Index   2(

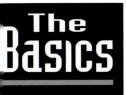

Abbreviations

BSA	bovine serum albumin
CFC	chlorofluorocarbon
CSS	cell suspension solution
DAB	diaminobenzidine
DAPI	4,6-diamidino-2-phenylindole
DC	dendritic cells
DMEM	Dulbecco's modified Eagle medium
ER	endoplasmic reticulum
EtBr	ethidium bromide
FCS	fetal calf serum
GBSS	Gey's balanced salt solution
HB	homogenization buffer
HDL	high-density lipoprotein
HIV	human immunodeficiency virus
HM	homogenization medium
HRP	horseradish peroxidase
Ig	immunoglobulin
LDL	low-density lipoprotein
LHM	lysosome homogenization medium
LRP	leukocyte-rich plasma
MS	microsome solution
NADPH	nicotinamide adenine dinucleotide (reduced)
PAGE	polyacrylamide gel electrophoresis
PB	protein buffer
PEG	polyethylene glycol
PHM	peroxisome homogenization medium
PMN	polymorphonuclear
PVP	polyvinylpyrrolidone
rAAV	recombinant adeno-associated virus
RCF	relative centrifugal field
RER	rough endoplasmic reticulum
rpm	revolutions per minute
RPMI	Roswell Park Memorial Institute medium
SDS	sodium dodecyl sulfate
SER	smooth endoplasmic reticulum
TBS	tricine-buffered saline
TGN	*trans* Golgi network
UDP	uridine diphosphate
UV	untraviolet

UWS	University of Wisconsin solution
VLDL	very low density lipoprotein
WGA	wheat-germ agglutinin
WS	working solution

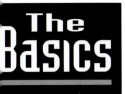

Preface

Although centrifugation is not regarded as an important modern technology in the same way as the techniques allied to studies of the human genome, proteomics and gene therapy, it does nevertheless underpin many of these new and exciting methods. Much of this technology still relies on an ability to purify cells, subcellular particles, viruses, proteins and nucleic acids efficiently and effectively; indeed in a recent survey of research workers at the US National Institutes of Health, over 65% replied that centrifugation was an integral part of their work. The first four chapters of this book are intended to provide the reader with a good working knowledge of how biological particles behave in a centrifugal field and how density gradients are used to fractionate them. They describe both the traditional centrifugation rotors and tubes and density gradient materials and their modern versions which permit easier sample handling and higher resolution of particles which retain more of their normal biological activity. An important aim of these chapters, which mix both theory and practice, is to help the reader to make the correct choice of centrifuge rotor, tube and gradient medium and select the most appropriate means of gradient making and collection.

Each of the final four chapters on the separation of mammalian cells, the major subcellular organelles, membrane vesicles and macromolecules and macromolecular complexes, provide a description of the strategies using both traditional and modern approaches. The subsequent detailed protocols cannot be anything approaching a comprehensive survey of the current technology and the selection probably reveals much about the author's own interests. Nevertheless, they should provide some important basic themes and pointers for the reader to apply to his or her own requirements.

John M Graham
email: john@jgrescon.fsbusiness.co.uk

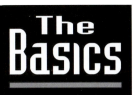

Chapter 1

Principles and strategies of centrifugation

1. Sedimentation of particles under the influence of gravity

The simple experiment many schoolchildren carry out to demonstrate the effect of gravity on a suspension of particles remains as instructive today as it always has. When a handful of soil and sand is shaken in a tall jar of water and then allowed to stand on the bench, large numbers of the particles immediately start to sediment to the bottom of the jar under the influence of the earth's gravitational field. The force on the particles is described as unit gravity or 1 g. When the sedimented material is examined after 10–15 min, several layers are observed; each layer consisting of particles of roughly the same size and generally, the size of the particles in the sediment increases from the top to the bottom (*Figure 1.1*). Some of the smaller particles in the water above the sediment are still moving slowly downwards, eventually (after 30–60 min) to form another layer, while others do not sediment at all, moving randomly around in the liquid phase and will never form a sedimented layer, even after several hours. When the experiment is repeated in a 20% solution of cane sugar, the process of sedimentation still occurs, but at a much slower rate and more particles remain in suspension.

The experiments demonstrates three important properties of all particles that sediment through a liquid in a centrifugal field:

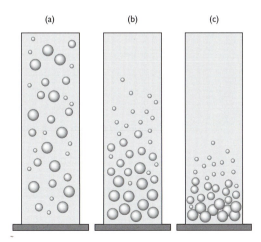

Figure 1.1

Time-dependent sedimentation at 1 g of particles in a liquid of uniform low density. (a) Particles randomly distributed at time zero; (b) particles sediment at a rate proportional to their size; (c) particle size in pellet increases top to bottom. Smallest particles remain in suspension.

- the rate of sedimentation of a particle depends on the diameter of the particle;
- a particle will only sediment into a stable pellet if the gravitational field can overcome the random thermal motion of the particle;
- the viscosity of the liquid retards the rate of sedimentation of all particles;
- the only other important particle parameter, not obvious from our simple experiment, is its density.

2.   Rate of sedimentation

One of the most useful equations (Equation 1.1) for the rate of sedimentation of a particle is derived from the Stokes equation, which describes the movement of a sphere through a liquid in a gravitational field. As the velocity of the sphere reaches a constant value, the net force on the sphere is equal to the force resisting its motion through the liquid (frictional drag).

$$\frac{1}{6}\pi d^3(\rho_p - \rho_l)g = 3\pi d\mu v \tag{1.1}$$

where, v = velocity of sedimentation; d = diameter of particle; ρ_p = density of particle; ρ_l = density of liquid; μ = viscosity of liquid; g = gravitational force.

This can be rearranged as Equation 1.2, one of the most widely quoted equations in centrifugation theory.

$$v = \frac{d^2(\rho_p - \rho_l)g}{18\mu}. \tag{1.2}$$

The behavior described by Equation 1.2 has some very important consequences, including:

- although v depends on the factor $(\rho_p - \rho_l)$, in a liquid of low uniform density, d^2 is generally the more important factor, except for very dense or very light particles;
- a particle will only sediment if $\rho_p > \rho_l$ and if $\rho_p < \rho_l$ then v will be negative and the particle will float up through the liquid rather than sediment.

These consequences are relevant to the three modes of preparative centrifugation – differential centrifugation (Section 4), rate-zonal sedimentation (Section 5.1) and buoyant density or equilibrium density banding (Section 5.2).

3.   Increasing the magnitude of the gravitational field

Although there are a few instances of the use of the earth's gravitational field (1 g) alone to effect a separation of biological particles (e.g. human blood cells will separate into layers of erythrocytes and leukocytes after standing on the bench for 1–2 h and mammalian cells of different sizes have been fractionated by allowing them to fall through a long liquid column), their small size requires the imposition of a much higher gravitational force. This is achieved by spinning a tube containing a suspension of the particles about an axis. The particles experience a radial centrifugal force moving them away from the axis of rotation. The machine which spins the tubes is called a centrifuge and the device that holds the tubes and rotates about the axis is called a rotor. Any particle, whether it is a cell or a macromolecule, is subjected to a centrifugal force when it is rotated at a certain speed and the centrifugal force (F) is expressed as in Equation 1.3:

$$F = m\omega^2 r \tag{1.3}$$

where F = magnitude of the centrifugal force; m = effective mass of the particle; ω = angular velocity (radians s^{-1}) and r = distance of the particle from the axis of rotation. Although Equation 1.3 is an important starting point for the derivation of the Svedberg equation (Section 6), the magnitude of the radial force generated by the spinning rotor is normally expressed relative to that of the earth's gravitational force and is known as the relative centrifugal field (RCF) or 'g force'. It is calculated according to Equation 1.4:

$$RCF = 11.18r \left(\frac{Q}{1000} \right)^2 \tag{1.4}$$

where Q = r.p.m. and r = distance of the particle from the axis of rotation (cm). This can be rearranged into a form for the calculation of Q required to produce a certain RCF (Equation 1.5).

$$Q = 299 \sqrt{\frac{RCF}{r}}. \tag{1.5}$$

The centrifugal force experienced by the particles thus depends on the rate of rotation and their distance from the axis of rotation. This equation has considerable significance when it comes to choice of rotor and selection of an appropriate value for Q (see Chapter 2).

Whether a particle in suspension is able to form a stable pellet depends not only on the g-force experienced by the particle, but the length of time for which it experiences this g-force; that is, the important factor is $g.t$. Moreover, as long as the imposed RCF is sufficient to overcome the random thermal motion of the particles, then if a particle sediments to form a stable pellet at 5000 g for 10 min, then the same result will be obtained at 2500 g for 20 min or 10 000 g for 5 min. Sometimes the conditions for sedimenting a particle are quoted in terms of $g.t$ (e.g. 50 000 g.min).

4. Differential centrifugation

The simplest form of fractionation by centrifugation is called differential centrifugation, a process sometimes called differential pelleting. A suspension of a mixed population of particles is subjected to a series of increasing $g.t$ values to produce a series of pellets containing particles of decreasing sedimentation rate. The most widely used application of this technique is to produce crude subcellular fractions from a tissue homogenate such as that from rat liver. The homogenate will contain nuclei, mitochondria, lysosomes, peroxisomes, sheets of plasma membrane and a huge spectrum of membrane vesicles derived from a variety of intracellular membrane compartments and also from the plasma membrane, normally in a buffered medium such as 0.25 M sucrose, 10 mM Tris–HCl, pH 7.4. The procedure is discussed in greater detail in Chapter 6 and the selection of the appropriate centrifuge rotor is considered in Chapter 2. Here the fractionation of an homogenate is merely used to illustrate the general strategy and efficacy of differential centrifugation as a separative technique.

If the homogenate is allowed to stand long enough, some of the larger and denser particles in the solution (principally the nuclei) will sediment to the bottom of the tube. However, most of the particles will never sediment significantly at 1 g, hence the use of a sequentially increasing g.t.

The homogenate is first centrifuged at 1000 g for 5–10 min, which is sufficient to pellet principally the nuclei – a consequence of their large size (and high density) as compared with the other subcellular particles. However, in centrifuging fast enough and long enough to pellet all the nuclei (many of which started off close to the top of the column of liquid and initially experienced the lowest RCF), more slowly moving particles, which started nearer the bottom of the tube (which only have to move a short distance and are exposed to the highest RCF), will also be found in the pellet. Reference to Equation 1.2 shows that, for particles of equal density, a large particle with a diameter of 5 μm will sediment four times faster than one with a diameter of 2.5 μm. In such cases then, all the smaller particles in the lower quarter of the centrifuge tube would sediment in the time taken for the larger particles, initially at the top of the tube, to pellet. Reducing the RCF may lessen this problem but then the recovery of the nuclei will also be reduced. See Chapter 2 for more information about the influence of rotor type on the efficiency of differential pelleting. There is an additional problem that arises simply from the physical entrapment of smaller particles during formation of the pellet.

In the differential centrifugation process, the 1000-g supernatant is then centrifuged at a higher g.t to pellet particles of the next lower order of size. This process of sequentially increasing the g.t is continued as many times as is necessary, although at least for a normal tissue homogenate, it is unusual to use more than four steps.

The problems of contamination and poor recoveries in differential centrifugation fractions are compounded by the heterogeneity in the size of any one type of biological particle. There is therefore no particular merit in increasing the number of steps and reducing the increment of the RCF in an attempt to improve the purity of the particles. With few exceptions the only result will be that each of the particle types will be distributed over a larger number of fractions. The microsomal pellet, which contains all of the membrane vesicles, is likely to be the purest fraction of the various differential centrifugation fractions of a tissue homogenate simply because of the large difference in particle size (*Table 1.1*) between that of most membrane vesicles and that of the next smallest group of particles (peroxisomes and lysosomes).

The problem of poor recoveries and contamination in differential centrifugation pellets is often addressed by repeating the centrifugation steps. For example, to recover more nuclei, the $5–10 \times 10^3$ g min^{-1} supernatant might be recentrifuged at the same RCF and time, while to remove some of

Table 1.1. Size of some subcellular organelles

Particle	d (μm)
Nuclei	4–12
Plasma membrane sheets	3–20
Mitochondria	0.4–2.5
Lysosomes	0.4–0.8
Peroxisomes	0.4–0.8
Vesicles	0.05–0.4

the smaller particles from the $5–10 \times 10^3$-g.min pellet, it may be resuspended in the homogenization medium and the centrifugation repeated. The latter procedure is often termed 'washing the pellet' and is sometimes extended to two or three washes. It can be an effective purification strategy, notably in the few cases where the d^2 value of the next largest particle is significantly less than that of the particle of interest. Nuclei and 'heavy mitochondria' (see Chapter 6) can be purified in this manner, by repeated washing of the appropriate pellets. Its disadvantages are that it is time consuming and resuspension of pellets, which requires the use of some sort of liquid shear force (usually a loose-fitting Dounce homogenizer), can lead to reduced yields and fragmentation of the particles. In most cases, however, to increase the purity of differential centrifugation fractions, one or more of the density gradient techniques that are discussed in Section 5 must be used.

Pelleting of cells, bacteria and viruses from large volumes of culture media is also used simply to concentrate the material prior to further analysis or continued culturing. This might be regarded as a limiting case of differential pelleting in which an RCF is chosen to sediment the particles while leaving the soluble nutrients in the supernatant. Virus cultures are often centrifuged first at 1000 g for 10 min to remove any cell debris (a process often called clarification) and the virus particles are then harvested at much higher RCFs (40 000–100 000 g)

In a few instances a pellet will exhibit an obvious stratification and if one or more of the upper layer can be resuspended by gentle agitation, this can provide a useful additional purification (see Chapter 6)

5.   Centrifugation in density gradients

It might be thought that if a suspension of particles was layered over a denser liquid, that a zone of particles would move down through the liquid at a rate that depended on their mass and size. However, as the particles must have a density greater than that of the liquid, the total density of the zone containing the particles will be greater than that of the liquid below it, hence the zone of particles will tumble down to the bottom of the tube; the zone is described as being unstable. This problem is avoided if the particle suspension is layered not over a liquid of uniform density but over a column of liquid whose density increases from top to bottom, that is, over a density gradient. The rise in concentration of solute molecules below the zone is able to compensate for the fall in the concentration of the particles in this region; under these conditions the zone is stable. The separation technique is called rate-zonal gradient centrifugation. The particles will continue to sediment as a zone through the gradient so long as the density of the surrounding liquid (ρ_l) is less than that of the particle (ρ_p). When $\rho_l = \rho_p$, the velocity of sedimentation will be zero (see Equation 1. 2), that is, the particle will have reached its equilibrium density (often called buoyant or isopycnic density) and stop moving.

In practice, gradients may either be continuous (i.e. the density increases in a smooth, but not necessarily linear fashion from top to bottom) or discontinuous (i.e. gradients are constructed from layers of increasing solute concentration whose density thus rises in step-like manner; *Figure 1.2*). See Chapter 4 for more information about making gradients.

5.1   Rate-zonal centrifugation strategies

In this technique, the sample is loaded as a narrow band on top of a continuous gradient of some suitable solute (e.g. sucrose). When centrifugation begins, the particles sediment through the gradient towards the bottom of the centrifuge tube as with differential centrifugation. As the particles in the band move down through the medium, the faster-sedimenting particles move ahead of the slower ones, so that a number of zones are formed, each containing particles of similar size and moving through the gradient at different rates (*Figure 1.3*). The distance between the zones increases with distance from the loading position, thus increasing the resolution between zones and the radial distance occupied by each zone depends on the volume of sample applied to the gradient. As with differential centrifugation, the speed at which the particles sediment depends principally on their size and to a smaller extent on their density and shape. The maximum density of the gradient must be less than the buoyant density of the particles being separated, otherwise sedimentation will terminate when $\rho_l = \rho_p$.

The gradient not only stabilizes the moving bands, but also provides a medium of increasing density and viscosity; both of these parameters gradually retard the sedimentation of the particles (Equation 1.2) while the increase in the RCF experienced by the particles in the spinning rotor accelerates them. In the ideal situation, these two opposing effects are balanced such that the zones of particles move down through the gradient at an approximately uniform rate. A density and viscosity range of the gradient should be chosen to conform as close as possible to this ideal situation (see

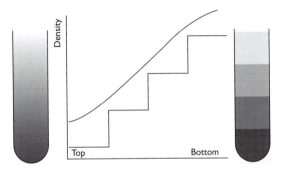

Figure 1.2

Density profiles of a continuous density gradient (left) and a discontinuous gradient (right).

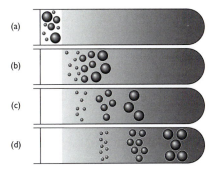

Figure 1.3

Rate-zonal (sedimentation velocity) of particles according to size in a continuous density gradient. (a) Suspension of particles layered on top of gradient; (b–d) particles move through gradient in centrifugal field in discrete zones.

below for an example). For this reason, discontinuous (layered) gradients in which there are sudden changes in density and viscosity are never used for rate-zonal work.

In rate-zonal centrifugation all the particles essentially start from approximately the same place, i.e. a narrow band on top of the gradient. Because the difference in RCF between the top and bottom of the sample layer is very small, compared to that in differential centrifugation (Section 4), the faster sedimenting species are not contaminated by the slower, as they are in differential centrifugation. On the other hand, the requirement for a narrow load zone limits the volume of sample that can be accommodated on one gradient, normally to approx 10% of the gradient volume.

Because the volume of sample that can be applied to a rate-zonal gradient is limited the concentration of particles in the sample tends to be high. However, because the rate of diffusion of particles and macromolecules in the sample is much lower than the rate of diffusion of the solute molecules from the top of the gradient into the sample, the density of the sample may exceed that of the top of the gradient leading to band broadening. In extreme cases this gradient instability leads to sedimentation of the sample in droplets (*Figure 1.4*). This situation is often described as exceeding the capacity of the gradient.

Band sharpening can be achieved by loading the sample in a medium of a viscosity much lower than that of the top of the gradient. When the sedimenting particles encounter the increased viscosity, their rate of sedimentation is slowed, allowing particles from the top of the low-viscosity sample zone to catch up.

■   Rate-zonal techniques are used principally if individual types of particles have different well-defined sizes and similar density that is much greater than that of even the densest part of the gradient.

■   If these conditions are met then the forces which are tending to retard the movement of the particle (the increasing viscosity of the gradient and the reduction in ($\rho_l - \rho_p$) are exactly balanced by the accelerating

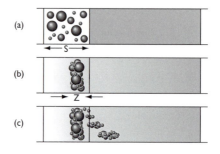

Figure 1.4

Instability of an interface between sample and gradient. (a) S = stable sample zone at time zero; (b) Under influence of centrifugal field, particles sediment rapidly into narrow zone (Z) while solute diffuses into S layer. Total density (solute + particles) of zone (Z) rises above that of the top of the gradient. (c) Droplets from (Z) zone fall through gradient.

force of the increasing RCF). **So the particles move through the gradient at a constant rate.** This ideal gradient situation is called isokinetic.

Thus it is for smaller, more slowly sedimenting, dense macromolecules and macromolecular complexes (proteins, nucleic acids, ribosomes, polysomes and ribosomal subunits) that rate-zonal density gradient centrifugation comes into its own. Ribosomes and ribosomal subunits, for example, are separated on the basis of their sedimentation rate in gradients of sucrose whose maximum density is no more than approx 1.2 g ml^{-1}. Since nucleic acids and ribosomes have densities in sucrose of at least 1.6 g ml^{-1}, and proteins of about 1.3 g ml^{-1}, the $(\rho_l - \rho_p)$ factor is never going to be significantly sedimentation rate-limiting (Chapter 8). The fractionation of proteins on the basis of molecular mass size in sucrose gradients is a widely used technique (Chapter 8).

One of the few examples of subcellular membranes that conform to these requirements is the sequence of compartments that are involved in the processing of macromolecules during endocytosis. The series of membrane-bound compartments that have similar densities but different sizes and the sequential modification of ligands can be analyzed in isoosmotic rate-zonal gradients (Chapter 7).

As a preparative technique for organelles, rate-zonal gradients have rather a limited application, not only because of the sample volume restriction, but also because of the heterogeneity of size of any one organelle type and the overlap of the size ranges of different organelles (*Table 1.1*). Generally these problems make the isolation of organelles by rate-zonal centrifugation rather less useful than one might expect. Moreover, when the particles also have different densities (*Table 1.2*), choice of density gradient and centrifugation conditions such that none of the particles reach their banding density $(\rho_l - \rho_p)$ may be very difficult to achieve. The only example worth quoting is that developed by Wisher and Evans (1975) for the purification of rat liver plasma membrane sheets from a 1000 g pellet.

When a suspension of the 1000 g pellet is layered over a sucrose gradient $(\rho = 1.06-1.25$ g ml$^{-1})$ and centrifuged at approximately 8000 g, the three

Table 1.2. Density (g ml⁻¹) of some organelles in sucrose

Organelle	ρ (g ml⁻¹)
Nuclei	>1.30
Plasma membrane sheets	1.14–1.19
Mitochondria	1.17–1.21
Lysosomes	1.19–1.21
Peroxisomes	1.18–1.23
Vesicles	1.06–1.26

major components, nuclei, plasma membrane sheets and mitochondria (in order of decreasing sedimentation rate), sediment as three distinct zones (*Figure 1.5*). Only the nuclei are capable of sedimenting through the entire gradient and only these particles are potentially capable of sedimenting at a more or less constant rate, at least through the top half of the gradient. Although they may be smaller than the plasma membrane sheets they sediment more rapidly because their density is much greater. As both the mitochondria and plasma membrane sheets approach the mid-point of the gradient, their $(\rho_l - \rho_p)$ factors decrease dramatically and there rate of sedimentation slows considerably. Thus although this is a rate-zonal separation, the density differences of the particles are a major factor. To achieve satisfactory resolution of the plasma membrane and mitochondria the centrifugation must be terminated when the plasma membrane reaches the midpoint of the gradient (*Figure 1.5*). Eventually the plasma membrane and the mitochondria will band at the same position as they both have approximately the same buoyant density (*Figure 1.5*).

■　In this gradient the increase in viscosity from the top to bottom of the gradient is approximately 10-fold, while the increase in RCF is unlikely to be more than threefold. To achieve ideal isokinetic rate-zonal conditions in a typical preparative gradient for organelles is thus virtually impossible.

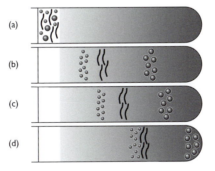

Figure 1.5

Fractionation of nuclei, plasma membrane and mitochondria in a continuous sucrose gradient. (a) Suspended nuclear pellet layered on top of gradient. During centrifugation at 8000 g for 40 min (b,c) nuclei (large circles), plasma membranes (lines) and mitochondria (small circles) sediment at rates proportional to their sizes. If centrifugation is continued for 2 h (d) the nuclei pellet and the mitochondria and plasma membranes band at the same buoyant density.

An additional problem, at least with sucrose gradients, is that since particles such as mitochondria and nuclei are osmotically active (they will lose water as they move through an increasingly hyperosmotic medium), their densities will increase to a limiting value and their size will reduce, making predictions about their behavior in a rate-zonal gradient very difficult. This can, however, be ameliorated by judicious choice of suitable gradient media (Chapter 3).

5.2   Isopycnic (buoyant density or equilibrium) separations

When centrifugation in a density gradient is carried out for a time that is sufficient to allow all the particles in the sample to reach that part of the gradient whose density is equivalent to that of the particles (i.e. where $\rho_l = \rho_p$ and $v = 0$), the gradient system is said to be isopycnic (from the Greek for density – *pyknos*) and the particles are separated according to their buoyant or banding density. The buoyant density of a particle is its apparent density in a liquid medium and this is measured as the density of the liquid at which $v = 0$ for the particle. Unlike the size of a biological particle, which can be measured independently by microscopy, the density of a biological particle can only be measured in the density gradient that is being used to prepare or analyze it. Since the density of many particles is sensitive to many factors, principally the osmotic pressure of the gradient, this parameter may vary significantly with the gradient medium that is being used (Chapter 3).

As with rate-zonal centrifugation the sample may be loaded on to a continuous density gradient, and the literature is full of such examples. In buoyant density fractionation, however, there is no absolute requirement for top loading: the sample can be placed in a dense medium at the bottom of the gradient (*Figure 1.6*), in which case the particles are in a medium of density greater than their own density, so $\rho_l < \rho_p$ and v will be negative; the particles will float up through the gradient (rather than sediment through it) until they reach their equilibrium position.

Provided buoyant density is the sole discriminating factor, the sample may even be distributed throughout the gradient (*Figure 1.6*). Irrespective of the size of the particles and their starting position in the gradient, all

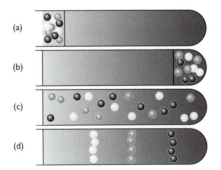

Figure 1.6

Buoyant density separation. Sample may be placed on top (a), beneath (b) or throughout density gradient (c). If centrifugation is carried out for a sufficient time, the particles will band at the same positions (d) irrespective of their starting point.

particles of the same density will band at the same position. For the same reason, the efficacy of the separation is not limited by the size of the sample.

A special and important case is the use of solutes (e.g. CsCl and iodix-anol) that form a gradient under the influence of the centrifugal field (self-generated, or self-forming) from a solution of uniform concentration (see Chapter 4). The sample is simply mixed with the medium and the gradient forms and the particles move to their buoyant density-banding positions during the centrifugation

Bottom loading the sample has considerable theoretical attractions, principally the avoidance of gradient overloading due to hydrodynamic instability of the sample/gradient interface (Section 5.1). Also, the contamination of particles by soluble proteins diffusing (and sedimenting) from the sample band is reduced by bottom loading, but may be more of a problem if the sample is distributed throughout the gradient. The disadvantage of bottom loading may be exposure to high concentrations of the gradient solute, although this will not be a problem with inert and isoosmotic solutes (see Chapter 3). More seriously, the sample will be exposed to the highest hydrostatic pressure, which may cause problems. There is evidence, for example, that mitochondria can be disrupted by high hydrostatic pressures (Wattiaux and Wattiaux-De Coninck, 1983). The magnitude of the hydrostatic pressure is proportional to the square of both the path-length of the tube and the rotor speed (see Chapter 2).

Band broadening can occur for a number of reasons; the use of too shallow a gradient (Section 5.1) and the heterogeneous nature of the particles may be contributive factors, but hydrostatic or hydrodynamic instability problems may also occur. Production of more than one band of apparently the same particle (*Figure 1.7*) may reflect the presence of two subpopulations or it may be caused by gradient instability. If the median section of particles

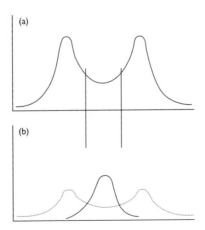

Figure 1.7

Artifactual banding. (a) Distribution of particles in a density gradient. (b) Particles within the median zone (between the two vertical lines) are recentrifuged in a second identical gradient. If the distribution in (a) is real, the particles will form a single band of median density (—); if artifactual, the original distribution will be repeated (....).

(between the two bands) is collected and re-run on a second gradient, the same biphasic profile will be produced if gradient stability is the problem but a true particle heterogeneity will result in a single band at the original position. A biphasic distribution may also be caused by gradient shape if the band is distributed across a shallow region between two steep gradients (see Chapter 4).

Unlike rate-zonal centrifugation, buoyant density-gradient centrifugation may be carried out in continuous or discontinuous gradients. Although a continuous gradient may provide a superior resolution and be more suited to an analytical purpose, for preparative purposes it may be beneficial to use a discontinuous gradient which has been designed so that one or more of the particles band in the sharp density gradient which is formed at the interface between layers. This often makes harvesting an easier job (see Chapter 4). In a discontinuous isopycnic gradient the sample may be incorporated into any or all of the layers.

If the discontinuous gradient comprises a single step, this is called a density barrier – it is often used to isolate one type of particle whose density is either greater or less than that of the barrier and greater or less (respectively) than that of all of the other particles. A rather special variation of this technique is the isolation of plasma lipoproteins by sequential flotation in which the lipoproteins of increasing density are allowed to float to the surface as the density of the plasma is raised in a step-like manner (see Chapter 8).

For more detailed accounts of the problems associated with the use of density gradients, see Dobrota and Hinton (1992)and Hinton and Mullock (1997).

6. Sedimentation coefficients and the Svedberg equation

The vast majority of centrifugation work today is aimed either at the preparation of biological particles or the analysis of subcellular processes. For such work, detailed information on the sedimenting characteristics of the particles, beyond a knowledge of their approximate density and the RCFs required either to sediment them or to band them in a gradient are not essential. Even studies of the interactions between macromolecules can be made without actual measurement of sedimentation velocities. Ultracentrifugation, however, was developed by the pioneering work of Svedberg and Pedersen (1940) as the one of the principal methods of determining the molecular mass of macromolecules, and although other methods such as gel electrophoresis have become more and more popular because of their ease of use, ultracentrifugation remains the gold standard method for this measurement. The use of ultracentrifugation was continued by workers such as Schumaker (1967) and Ifft (1969) to provide information on sedimentation coefficients, solvation and molecular interactions of proteins. It is beyond the scope of this introductory text to do more than present a couple of the most important aspects of the mathematical treatment of particle sedimentation.

The sedimentation rate of a particle per unit of centrifugal force is the sedimentation coefficient and it is described by Equation 1.6.

$$v = \frac{dr}{dt} = s\omega^2 r \qquad (1.6)$$

In Equation 1.6 dr/dt is the rate of movement of the particle (cm s^{-1}) and s is the sedimentation coefficient. Commonly, s is defined under standard conditions with water as the solvent at 20°C and is expressed as $s_{20,w}$. Sedimentation coefficients have units of seconds and as most macromolecules have an s value of 10^{-13} – 10^{-11} s, it is normal practice to express these values as Svedberg units (S), where $1S = 1 \times 10^{-13}$ S. The s value is often used to describe biological particles; indeed, all such particles can be described in this manner, but only macromolecules (proteins and nucleic acids) and some macromolecular complexes (such as ribosomes and ribosomal subunits) are routinely defined in this manner. Nevertheless, it is instructive to compare the sedimentation coefficients of a range of biological particles (*Figure 1.8*); thus proteins have sedimentation coefficients between 1 and 10S and nucleic acids 30 and 50S, while the sedimentation coefficient of a particle such as a mitochondrion is approx 10 000 times greater than a soluble protein. Moreover, there are software programs that permit the derivation of the appropriate gradient centrifugation conditions for the separation of a particle of known s-value (Young, 1984).

The molecular mass (M) of a particle can be computed from the famous Svedberg equation (Equation 1.7), which relates M to the diffusion coefficient of the molecule (D), its sedimentation coefficient, the density the liquid (ρ), the partial specific volume of the particle ($\bar{v}$), which is equivalent to the reciprocal of the particle density ($1/\rho_p$), R and T.

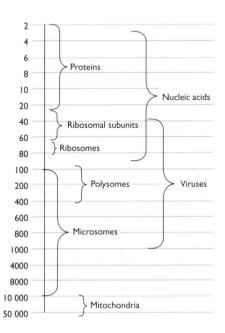

Figure 1.8

Sedimentation coefficients of biological particles. Figures on vertical scale are $s_{20,w}$.

$$M = \frac{RTs}{D(1 - \bar{v}\rho)} \tag{1.7}$$

Because diffusion coefficients of macromolecules are difficult to measure, however, the equation is of limited use. The Svedberg equation applies to a situation in which the particles are centrifuged at a sufficiently high centrifugal force to sediment them. A more useful situation is one in which the force causes the particles to sediment until they reach an equilibrium position where the centrifugal force is exactly balanced by the frictional force opposing their movement. This is measurement of molecular mass by sedimentation equilibrium. The molecular mass is then calculated from the following equation (Equation 1.8):

$$M = \frac{RT}{(1 - \bar{v}\rho)\omega^2}\left(\frac{1}{rc}\right)\left(\frac{dc}{dr}\right) \tag{1.8}$$

where dc/dr is the change in concentration of particles (c) as a function of distance from the axis of the rotor (r).

For up-to-date treatments of the theory of analytical centrifugation, see Rickwood (1984), Eason (1984), Spragg and Steensgard (1992) and Steensgard *et al.* (1992).

References

Dobrota, M. and Hinton, R. (1992) Conditions for density gradient separations. In: *Preparative Centrifugation – A Practical Approach* (ed. D. Rickwood). IRL Press a Oxford University Press, Oxford, pp. 77–142.

Eason, R. (1984) Analytical ultracentrifugation. In: *Centrifugation – A Practical Approach* (ed. D. Rickwood). IRL Press at Oxford University Press, Oxford, pp 251–286.

Hinton, R.H. and Mullock, B.M. (1997) Isolation of subcellular fractions. In: *Subcellular Fractionation – A Practical Approach* (eds J.M. Graham and D Rickwood). IRL Press at Oxford University Press, Oxford, pp. 31–69.

Ifft, J.B. (1969) Proteins at sedimentation equilibrium in density gradients. In: *A Laboratory Manual of Analytical Methods of Protein Chemistry*, Vol. 5 (ed P. Alexander and H.P. Lundgren). Pergamon Press, Oxford, pp. 151–223.

Rickwood, D. (1984) The theory and practice of centrifugation. In: *Centrifugation – A Practical Approach* (ed. D. Rickwood). IRL Press at Oxford University Press Oxford, pp. 1–43.

Schumaker, V.N. (1967) Zone centrifugation. *Adv. Biol. Med. Phys.* **11**: 245–339.

Spragg, S.P. and Steensgard, J. (1992) Theoretical aspects of practical centrifugation In: *Preparative Centrifugation – A Practical Approach* (ed. D. Rickwood). IRL Press at Oxford University Press, Oxford, pp. 1–42.

Steensgard, J., Humphries, S. and Spragg, S.P. (1992) Measurement of sedimentation coefficients. In: *Preparative Centrifugation – A Practical Approach* (ed D. Rickwood). IRL Press at Oxford University Press, Oxford, pp. 187–232.

Svedberg, T. and Pedersen, K.O. (1940) *The Ultracentrifuge.* The Clarendon Press Oxford.

Wattiaux, R. and Wattiaux-De Coninck S. (1983) Separation of cell organelles. In: *Iodinated Density Gradient Media – A Practical Approach* (ed. D. Rickwood). IRL Press at Oxford University Press, Oxford, pp. 119–137.

Wisher, M. H. and Evans, W.H. (1975) Functional polarity of the rat hepatocyte surface membrane. *Biochem. J.* **146**: 375–388.

Young, B.D. (1984) Measurement of sedimentation coefficients and computer simulation of rate-zonal separations. In: *Centrifugation – A Practical Approach* (ed D. Rickwood). IRL Press at Oxford University Press, Oxford, pp. 127–159.

Chapter 2

Centrifugation hardware

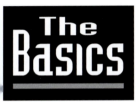

This chapter presents the range of hardware (centrifuges, rotors and tubes) which is currently available, describes good centrifuge practice for the general handling of rotors and tubes and discusses the relation between rotor type and the applications to which each rotor is most suited.

1. Centrifuges – an overview

Centrifuges are traditionally classified into three groups according to the maximum speed they can achieve. Low-speed centrifuges generally have a maximum speed up to 7000 r.p.m. (maximum relative centrifugal field, RCF, approximately 8000 g), high-speed centrifuges – up to 21 000 r.p.m. (maximum RCF approximately 40 000–50 000 g) and ultracentrifuges above 21 000 r.p.m. Over the years engineering developments have allowed the maximum speed of ultracentrifuges to increase from 50 000 r.p.m. to 150 000 r.p.m. (generating maximum RCFs of almost 1 000 000 g). The relation between r.p.m. and RCF in different rotors is described in Section 5.

Advances in engineering technology have allowed the introduction of direct drive systems, microchip processing for automated operation, the design of more compact models and the development of solid-state cooling systems, which eliminate the need for environmentally damaging chloroflu-orocarbons (CFCs) and compressors.

Older machines only operated at a single rate of acceleration which depended not only on the motor itself but also the mass of the rotor. Deceleration could be performed either with or without the brake. Although fast acceleration and deceleration rates are often presented by centrifuge manufacturing companies as important selling points, there is often a need to provide controlled slow acceleration or deceleration, particularly over the range 0–5000 r.p.m. Reorientation of gradients in tubes of fixed-angle rotors requires slow and smooth acceleration and deceleration. Rapid changes in r.p.m. can lead to the production of vortices in the liquid (Coriolis effect) with consequent mixing of the sample. Simple pelleting of particles tends to be less affected by these problems, although the effect can be seen when whole blood is centrifuged to pellet the erythrocytes which are seen to swirl up into the plasma supernatant if the rotor comes to rest suddenly. Modern high-speed and ultracentrifuges provide a series of controlled acceleration and deceleration programs; some low-speed centrifuges provide a similar facility, albeit on a less sophisticated scale.

The latest high-speed and ultracentrifuges also permit the operator to key in the rotor type being used. Not only can this provide a useful means of logging the rotor's total spinning time, it also allows the rotor speed indicator not only to provide the routine rotational speed in r.p.m. but also of the

RCF generated in that particular rotor. Many ultracentrifuges also allow computation of the rotor speed as an angular velocity in radians s^{-1} (ω).

While some low-speed centrifuges are still available in an unrefrigerated mode, it has become common practice for all centrifuges that are used for the processing of biological particles to be refrigerated. Heat is generated by friction in the spinning rotor and produced by the motor, hence there is a tendency for the temperature of the rotor (and the sample) to rise with time. Although low-speed centrifuges are used principally for the purification of cells at an unspecified room temperature, there are several standard density-gradient barrier methods for the isolation of leukocyte fractions from human blood that are only effective within a narrow temperature range (20–22°C). Thus, although low temperatures may not be necessary, good temperature control is still required, so an effective adjustable cooling device is now more of a routine feature.

In the case of all other centrifuges (high-speed and ultra) refrigeration is a prerequisite because of the increased heat generation at the higher speeds of these machines and these are frequently used for prolonged periods in which the sample must be maintained at 0–4°C. In addition, the rotor chamber of all ultracentrifuges is operated under vacuum to reduce the heat of friction further. Swinging-bucket type rotors generate more frictional heat than do angle rotors unless they are wind-shielded. Temperatures in all centrifuges can usually be controlled over the range -10 to $+40$°C.

There have been several major developments in centrifugation engineering over the last couple of decades which have blurred the classification of centrifuges on the basis of speed and changed the traditional view that all high-speed and ultracentrifuges had to be 'big'. There has been a major proliferation of bench-top varieties of high-speed centrifuges, many of which replace the need for a separate low-speed model. These have maximum speeds of 5000–20 000 r.p.m. There is also a type of high-speed centrifuge (Sorvall Supraspeed™) which is capable of speeds of up to 28 000 r.p.m. providing RCFs of up to 100 000g (against the 40 000–50 000g of most high-speed centrifuges), although only the smaller volume fixed-angle rotors are capable of running at the highest speeds. In these machines those rotors running at the highest speeds are run in a vacuum and they are therefore similar to a 'low-speed' ultracentrifuge in this respect.

Microcentrifuges are specially designed bench-top models which have light, small-volume rotors which are capable of very rapid acceleration up to approximately 17 000 r.p.m. They are compact machines which are usually (but not always) unrefrigerated and are principally used for short-time centrifugation of samples up to about 2 ml. Because of their small size, however, they are easily transportable and can be operated in a cold-room if necessary.

The new microultracentrifuges are specially designed to maximize centrifugation efficiency by permitting the use of small volume samples (normally of no more than 2–4 ml) at speeds of up to 100 000–150 000 r.p.m. By using small volume samples, very high RCFs (up to approximately 800 000g) and the latest rotor technology separations, which might have taken up to 16 h in larger volume, slower rotors, can now be carried out in a fraction of the time. These machines are either bench-top or floor-standing, and both are a fraction of the weight and dimensions of a standard floor-standing ultracentrifuge.

2. Basic rotor design

There are essentially only two designs of centrifuge rotor, swinging-bucket and fixed-angle, in general use. Although there is a great diversity of operational design, in all swinging-bucket rotors the centrifuge tube is accommodated in a pivoted bucket which rotates from a vertical to a horizontal position during acceleration, under the influence of the radial centrifugal field (*Figure 2.1a*). In this mode the meniscus of the sample always remains at right-angles to the axis of the tube. On the other hand the fixed-angle rotor accommodates the tube in a pocket within the body of the rotor maintaining the tube at the same angle to the vertical axis of the rotor at rest and during rotation. In such a rotor, the meniscus of the liquid rotates from a horizontal to a vertical plane during acceleration under the influence of the centrifugal field (*Figure 2.1b*). The basic design of the fixed-angle rotor is essentially similar in all types of centrifuge; the only important operational consideration is the angle of the tube to the vertical axis. This can be as high as 45° and as low as 18°, although there are two variants of this design in which the tube angle is approximately 8° (near-vertical rotor) or 0° (vertical rotor); these are discussed further in Section 5. The angle of the tube has important implications for formation of particle pellets (Section 8.1) and the sedimentation path-length of the rotor (Section 5).

The rotors of all centrifuges, but particularly those of ultracentrifuges, have to withstand considerable stress. Rotors for high-speed centrifuges and those for ultracentrifuges capable of speeds up to approximately 40 000 r.p.m.

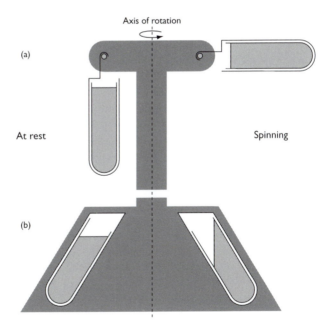

Figure 2.1

Comparison of swinging-bucket (a) and fixed-angle rotor (b). The meniscus of the liquid in the swinging-bucket tube is always at right angles to the axis of tube. In the fixed-angle rotor the meniscus reorients in the tube during acceleration.

have generally been constructed from aluminum, but most higher-speed rotors are made from titanium. There has been a move over recent years to try to reduce the mass of some of the largest volume high-speed fixed-angle rotors, and lightweight carbon-fiber rotors for ultracentrifuges have been introduced in order to make them easier to handle and to reduce the load imposed on the centrifuge drive system.

3. Rotor capacity and performance

From purely dimensional considerations, the floor-standing models can generally accommodate larger sample volumes than the bench-top models; they are also able to offer a larger range of tube volumes (and tube numbers) than can the bench-top models which are usually restricted to smaller-volume rotors. Generally speaking, the maximum speed of any centrifuge can only be achieved by the smaller-volume fixed-angle rotors while the larger-volume rotors (particularly the swinging-bucket rotors) have reduced maximum speeds.

Large-volume rotors, especially, offer the use of smaller-volume tubes through the use of plastic adaptors which fit into the rotor bucket (swinging-bucket) or rotor pocket (fixed-angle) and effectively reduce its usable volume. With the largest-volume swinging-bucket rotors in particular, the adaptor often permits the use of two or more of the smaller-volume tubes in each bucket. With low-speed and high-speed centrifuges, the use of adaptors rarely compromises the permitted maximum speed of the rotor, while with ultracentrifuges the extreme stresses often impose a reduction in the maximum r.p.m. Routinely, adaptors reduce the diameter of the tube space, while the g-Max® adaptors produced by Beckman, which reduce the length of the tube, are used only for special purposes (Section 8.2).

Low-speed centrifuges of the large, floor-standing type, will accept up to 6×1 l, while the medium-sized models will take up to 4×500 ml samples and the bench-top models 4×250 ml. In general, low-speed centrifuges use the swinging-bucket type rotor and may have interchangeable rotor heads to accept buckets of different capacities. Routinely, it is more likely for a multi-user machine to be equipped with a rotor carrying large-capacity buckets that can be adapted to take larger numbers of smaller-volume tubes.

Floor-standing high-speed centrifuges normally have a maximum capacity of 6×500 ml and bench-top models can accommodate 8×15 ml or 4×50 ml, with some able to take 6×100 ml. The majority of the bench-top models are aimed at the small-volume sample (1–50 ml).

Floor-standing ultracentrifuges have a maximum capacity of 6×100 ml, with the larger-volume rotors having a severe restriction on the maximum rotor-speed, sometimes as low as 20 000 r.p.m. The majority of applications use rotors with 5–50 ml capacity. Although microultracentrifuges are specifically designed for small (1–4 ml) samples, some rotors may accommodate tubes with volume of up to 8 ml but again these and swinging-bucket rotors have significant speed restrictions.

Note that rotor capacities given by centrifuge companies (e.g. 8×15 ml) indicate only the maximum capacity for each tube; in most cases, the actual volume of the tube depends upon the wall thickness of the tube and the useful volume is usually 5–10% less than that quoted.

Detailed specifications of a large selection of ultracentrifuge rotors are given in Rickwood (1992a).

4. Uses of centrifuges and rotors

It is necessary to make a distinction between the use of centrifuges and centrifuge rotors for (a) harvesting of particles from culture media, homogenates and cell extracts, in which the selection of the appropriate centrifuge and rotor depends almost solely on the rate of sedimentation of the particles and (b) the subsequent purification or analysis of particles using density gradients which generally require much higher RCFs than those needed for simple pelleting.

Generally speaking, intact cells are centrifuged at room temperature; this is particularly the case if centrifugation is part of a continuous cell culture process. As most mammalian cells are grown at $37°C$ and bacteria often at room temperature, it serves no useful purpose to carry out centrifugation at $4°C$, indeed, it may actually be detrimental to some mammalian cells. Low-temperature centrifugation is only necessary when any subsequent analysis requires the cell metabolism to be arrested or the cells are to be used for the preparation of subcellular organelles or macromolecules. Most other separations are carried out at $4°C$ to reduce potential enzymic breakdown of macromolecules, although there are exceptions; plasma lipoproteins for instance have routinely been separated at $16°C$.

Low-speed centrifuges are used to harvest chemical precipitates, intact cells (animal, plant and some microorganisms), nuclei, chloroplasts, large mitochondria and the larger plasma-membrane fragments. Density gradients for purifying cells are also run in these centrifuges. Swinging-bucket rotors tend to be used very widely because of the huge flexibility of sample size through the use of adaptors (see manufacturer's literature for details).

High-speed centrifuges are used to harvest some microorganisms, viruses, mitochondria, lysosomes, peroxisomes and intact tubular Golgi membranes. The majority of the simple pelleting tasks are carried out in fixed-angle rotors. Some density-gradient work for purifying cells and organelles can be carried out in swinging-bucket rotors, or in the case of Percoll gradients (Chapter 4) in fixed-angle rotors

Ultracentrifuges are used to harvest all membrane vesicles derived from the plasma membrane, endoplasmic reticulum (ER) and Golgi membrane, endosomes, ribosomes, ribosomal subunits, plasmids, DNA, RNA and proteins in fixed-angle rotors. They are the most commonly used centrifuge for the density-gradient purification of all particles except cells, and while swinging buckets have been traditionally used for this purpose, fixed-angle rotors and vertical rotors are also used, particularly for self-generated gradients (Chapter 4) and can improve the efficiency of separation greatly.

5. Centrifuge rotor parameters

Rotors are routinely described by their type: swinging-bucket, fixed-angle, vertical or near-vertical; by their sample volume capacity and the number of tubes (of the maximum volume), and by their maximum speed (in r.p.m). Often the maximum volume per tube is a nominal value which is approximately the usable volume of the tube pocket or bucket. The actual tube volume will depend on the tube type – the thickness of its wall and whether it is open-topped, capped or sealed (Section 6). Moreover, the bucket or tube pocket of many rotors can be adapted to accommodate smaller volume tubes and those of larger volume rotors (for many low-speed and high-speed centrifuges but rather rarely for ultracentrifuges) often have adaptors for multiple tubes of smaller volumes. Consult the manufacturer's literature for details.

In a swinging-bucket rotor the geometry of the tube space (*Figure 2.2a*) is described in terms of the distance from the axis of the rotor to the top of the tube (r_{max}), to the midpoint of the long axis (r_{av}) and to the bottom of the tube (r_{max}). In the case of fixed-angle rotors, the angle at which the tube his held influences these values (*Figure 2.2b*), so that r_{min} is more accurately described as the distance from the axis to the inner wall of the tube at its nearest point to the axis, and r_{max} is the distance from the axis to the inner wall of the tube at its furthest point from the axis. The same is true for the near-vertical rotor (*Figure 2.2c*). The vertical rotor is the limiting case in which the three values are measured across the diameter of the tube (*Figure 2.2d*).

The RCF values are also measured at these three points to provide g_{min} *etcetera*. Without exception, the RCF generated by the rotor at its maximum speed is quoted by manufacturers as the g_{max}, that is, the RCF at the r_{max} of

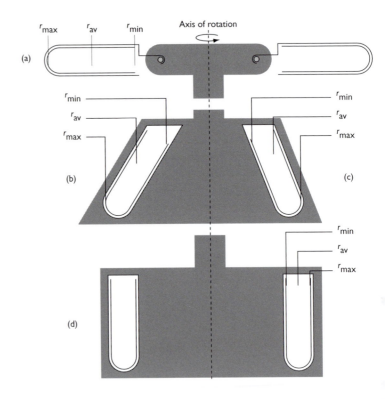

Figure 2.2

Comparison of r values of rotors. Swinging-bucket (a), fixed-angle (b), near-vertical (c) and vertical (d) rotors.

the tube. This is not a particularly useful concept. In most experimental protocols, the required RCF is quoted in terms of the g_{av}. It is a more useful description of the RCF experienced by the sample when it fills the tube. In tubes which are only partially filled, it is more relevant to consider the g_{av} at the midpoint of the sample, which will be higher than the g_{av} of the tube, while the g_{max} will not change. The following equations are used to convert r.p.m. (Q) to RCF and vice versa.

$$RCF = 11.18r\left(\frac{Q}{1000}\right)^2 \tag{2.1}$$

$$Q = 299\sqrt{\frac{RCF}{r}}_2 \tag{2.2}$$

where r is the radial distance in centimeters.

A few worked examples that show the difference in RCF at r_{max}, r_{av} and r_{min} between different rotors are given in *Table 2.1*. The top three are commonly used ultracentrifuge rotors while the bottom three are microultracentrifuge rotors. The increase in RCF between r_{min} and r_{max} varies from as little as 24% for the VTi65.1 (vertical) to 128% for the SW41Ti (swinging-bucket), while for the 70.1Ti (fixed-angle) the value is 102%. The TLA100.2, TLN100 and TLA120.1 rotors are capable of much higher r.p.m.s but have considerably smaller r values.

The difference between the r_{max} and the r_{min} is called the sedimentation path-length of the tube and is a very important parameter when considering the efficiency of sedimentation of particles both through a solution of uniform density and through a gradient (Sections 8 and 9) and for the formation of self-generated gradients (Chapter 4).

6. Centrifuge tubes

There is a huge range of centrifuge tube types and tube materials for each class of centrifuge and it is not feasible to give more than a brief overview here.

Table 2.1. RCF values at r_{min}, r_{av} and r_{max} for selected Beckman–Coulter ultracentrifuge rotors[a]

Rotor	Type[b]	Tube (ml)	Q (r.p.m.)	r_{min}	r_{av}	r_{max}	g_{min}	g_{av}	g_{max}
SW41 Ti	SW	14	40 000	6.74	11.02	15.31	120 565	197 125	273 865
70.1 Ti	FA	13.5	60 000	4.05	6.12	8.20	163 000	246 320	330 035
VTi65.1	V	13.5	60 000	6.85	7.67	8.49	275 700	308 700	341 705
TLA100.2	FA	2.0	100 000	2.45	3.18	3.89	273 910	355 525	434 900
TLN100	NV	3.9	100 000	2.31	3.16	4.02	258 260	353 290	449 435
TLA120.1	FA	0.5	120 000	2.45	3.18	3.89	394 430	511 655	626 260

r values in cm.
SW, swinging-bucket; FA, fixed-angle; NV, near-vertical; V, vertical.

6.1   Materials

Glass centrifuge tubes are still commonly used for low-speed centrifugation but with the exception of use for work with organic solvents, most operations can be more conveniently carried out in plastic tubes. Ordinary Pyrex glass tubes can withstand forces of around 2000 g, while Corex® glass tubes can be centrifuged at up to 12 000 g. Plastic tubes have the advantage of cheapness and can be obtained ready-sterilized (an important consideration for harvesting cultured cells). Polyethylene, polyallomer and polypropylene are the most commonly used plastics; the main disadvantage of some types is their relative opacity compared with glass. Polycarbonate tubes tend to be more expensive but they are more or less transparent. Polycarbonate and polyallomer are the most commonly used materials for high-speed and ultracentrifuge tubes, with polypropylene being rather less common.

Choice of a particular tube material can be a simple case of personal preference, but there may be factors to be considered relating to the possible reactivity of the tube material and the maximum RCF which it is designed to withstand. If samples are likely to contain organic solvents, it is imperative that manufacturer's specifications are consulted before using a particular type of tube. Glass is the most obvious choice for solvent resistance but plastic tubes do have some restricted solvent resistance. In general, polycarbonate is least resistant and polyallomer most resistant to organic solvents. All plastic tubes can be used with any aqueous materials but there may be some special requirements posed by specific biological particles. For example, monocytes tend to adhere to plastic surfaces, and polypropylene is particularly prone to this problem. Of the synthetic materials, only cellulose proprionate cannot be autoclaved, but this is one of the few synthetics that can be sterilized by ultraviolet (UV) radiation. In the authors' experience repeated autoclaving of polycarbonate tubes leads to stress damage, which in turn may lead to breakage during centrifugation. The manufacturer provide extensive information with regard to solvent, salt and pH resistance and provide sterilization procedures for centrifuge tubes; this information has also been summarized by Rickwood (1992b).

Clear plastics such as polycarbonate and polyethylene terephthalate and some of the trade-marked materials such as Ultraclear® and Polyclear® make visualization of banded material in gradients more easy than the more opaque materials such as polyallomer.

6.2   Tubes for low-speed and high-speed rotors

For the sedimentation of intact cells in low-speed centrifuges, it is necessary to use the minimum force required to obtain a pellet which is not too compact. A very compact pellet of cells leads to cell damage and loss of function or recovery. It is therefore advisable to use a conical-bottomed centrifuge tube in a swinging-bucket rotor, as the conical-shaped bottom retains the pellet more effectively as the supernatant is removed. The pellet is also more securely held against the liquid vortex, which may occur if the rotor slows from maximum speed to rest too quickly.

The tubes for low-speed and high-speed centrifuges are rather similar in that they tend to be thick walled and available in either an open-topped or simple screw-cap varieties. Tubes with snap-on caps are also available. Rather better containment is offered by tubes which are closed by a central plastic plug and O-ring which is sealed on to the top of the tube neck by a screw-cap. The choice of tube type depends on both personal preference and the type of material being processed.

The conical-bottomed or round-bottomed screw-cap plastic tubes (10, 12, 15 and 50 ml) which are widely used and widely available from general laboratory and tissue culture plasticware companies are the 'work-horses' of low-speed centrifugation. They provide an acceptable level of containment for the handling of most samples from experimental animals and also human blood samples from volunteers within a laboratory who have been tested for antibodies to human imunodeficiency virus (HIV) and hepatitis. Potentially pathogenic or toxic material should only be used in tubes which offer the highest degree of containment. The buckets of some swinging-bucket rotors for these centrifuges are now available with screw-on sealed domes to provide extra containment.

6.3   Tubes for ultracentrifuge rotors

Tubes for ultracentrifuges are rather more specialized because of the extra stress imposed on them. Thick-walled polycarbonate or polyallomer tubes, either with a central plug, O-ring and screw-cap (*Figure 2.3*) or open top are available. For the higher performance rotors, thick-walled tubes may have a restriction of the maximum permitted r.p.m. Thick-walled tubes, however, are the only ultracentrifuge tubes that can be run partially filled. All other thin-walled tubes in fixed-angle rotors must be completely filled and those in swinging-bucket rotors filled to within 3 mm of the top, otherwise they will tend to collapse under the stress of the radial centrifugal field. Swinging-bucket rotors are used almost exclusively with thin-walled tubes (although there are one or two thick-walled examples); they are never capped, the screw lid of the bucket providing the necessary seal. Vertical and near-vertical rotors only use thin-walled sealed tubes (see below).

Thin-walled tubes are made principally of polyallomer, although Beckman-Coulter Inc. produces a tube called 'Ultraclear®', which has the transparency of polycarbonate. Polyethylene terephthalate Polyclear® tubes

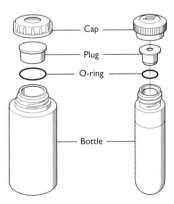

Cap

Plug

O-ring

Bottle

Figure 2.3

Exploded view of thick-walled ultracentrifuge tubes with screw-caps, incorporating central sealing plug. Reproduced from H. Roth and D. Rickwood (1992) Centrifuges and rotors. In: Preparative Centrifugation – a Practical Approach *(ed D. Rickwood). IRL Press at Oxford University Press. With permission of Oxford University Press.*

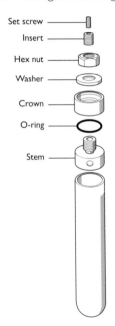

Set screw

Insert

Hex nut

Washer

Crown

O-ring

Stem

Figure 2.4

Exploded view of multiple-part cap for thin-walled ultracentrifuge tube. With the insert firmly screwed into the stem, the bottom five components are loosely assembled and fitted over the partly filled tube. The hex-nut is tightened and the tube completely filled with liquid from a syringe before the set screw is positioned to seal the tube.

(Sorvall Instruments) have a similar transparency. Bands of material in density gradients can be more readily visualized in these tubes but tube puncture (Chapter 4), although possible, is more difficult than with a polyallomer tube.

To achieve complete sealing of thin-walled tubes for fixed-angle (not vertical or near-vertical) rotors, one solution is to use multiple part caps (*Figure 2.4*), which when assembled on the tube allow complete filling (from a syringe) through a small central channel, which is subsequently sealed by a set-screw (or sealing-screw).

Sealed tubes

The more modern approach is to use tubes sealed either by heat, by crimping or by some form of plastic plug. The tops of these and other sealed tubes require support by a cap or spacer. Sealed tubes are used to advantage with potentially hazardous samples and are always used with near-vertical and vertical rotors.

With heat-sealed tubes a small metal cap is placed on the narrow neck of the tube which is melted by applying a hot iron (the Beckman–Coulter Tube Topper®) to the cap under pressure (*Figure 2.5a*). The top is subsequently cooled rapidly by applying a metal rod as a heat sink. The method is rapid but not entirely foolproof since, in the interval between removal of the hot iron and applying the heat sink, the melted top may deform slightly.

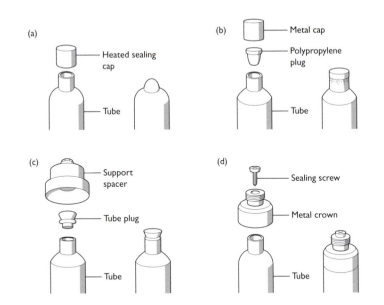

Figure 2.5

Sealed tubes. (a) A metal sealing cap is placed over Beckman Quickseal™ tubes and the plastic neck is sealed under pressure by applying a hot iron to the metal cap. (b) Sorvall Crimpseal™ tubes have a plastic plug covered by a metal cap that is mechanically compressed onto the tube neck. (c) The central plug of Beckman Optiseal™ tubes is sealed into the neck by pressure from the rotor pocket hex-nut on the support spacer. (d) The crown of Sorvall Re-seal™ tubes has a central plastic core that is expanded into the neck by a central sealing screw. Reproduced from H. Roth and D. Rickwood (1992) Centrifuges and rotors. In: Preparative Centrifugation – a Practical Approach (ed D. Rickwood). IRL Press at Oxford University Press. With permission of Oxford University Press.

Crimp-sealed (*Figure 2.5b*) tubes are closed with a plastic plug which is then crimped within a metal cap by a mechanical crimper (Sorvall Instruments). In the authors' hands the method is rather more reliable than heat-sealing.

Sealed tubes are most commonly made from polyallomer but both Beckman–Coulter and Sorvall provide these sealed tubes in the transparent Ultraclear® or polyethylene terephthalate, respectively.

While providing excellent sealing properties, neither of these tube types can be readily unloaded by upward displacement since this requires a flat tube top in order to make a seal with the unloading device, and unloading from the bottom by aspiration (Chapter 4) requires the use of a razor blade or scalpel to remove the sealed top (neither of which are to be recommended). Some form of tube puncture (Chapter 4) is the recommended method. The most recent types of sealed tubes allow easier access to the top of the tube since it is not irreversibly sealed.

In Optiseal® tubes (Beckman–Coulter), the neck is simply sealed under pressure with a plastic plug and O-ring (*Figure 2.5c*). In Re-seal® and Easyseal® tubes (Sorvall Instruments), although there are differences in detail of usage, both involve some form of external support in the form of a cap or collar and a central sealing plug which is screwed into the neck while the tube is immobilized in a vise (*Figure 2.5d*).

In these three types of tube, access to the top of the tube after centrifugation can be achieved simply by removing the central plug. Although Optiseal® tubes are the easiest to seal and unseal, the very flat shoulders of these tubes can cause loss of resolution during unloading by upward displacement; particles close the wall of the tube can become lodged just under the shoulder. Re-seal® and Easyseal® tubes on the other hand have rounded or conical tops and provide a better configuration for upward displacement.

7.   Good tube and rotor practice

7.1 Loading tubes and rotors

Rotors for the high-speed and ultracentrifuges are subjected to high stresses and precise balance of the rotors and the sample tubes they contain is absolutely essential. While balance is important for all rotors, those used in high-speed and ultracentrifuges will not tolerate the sometimes careless handling given to the low-speed versions. In all rotors, the centrifuge tubes used must be balanced to within the limits set by the manufacturer, usually within 0.1 g. Tubes placed in diametrically opposed positions must contain not only the same weight but also the same volume of liquid, that is they must contain liquid of the same density; only then will the center of gravity of the two tubes be the same and the center of gravity of the rotor will not be altered when they are added to the rotor – the rotor is said to be dynamically balanced. Tubes must not be overfilled; this is particularly important for uncapped tubes in fixed-angle rotors because the meniscus reorients within the tube during acceleration (*Figure 2.1*), and overfilled tubes are likely to lead to spillage and imbalance of the rotor. Tubes containing density gradients must be balanced by tubes containing exactly the same gradients in any rotor, although it is common practice for the low-density gradients usually used for cell separations in low-speed centrifuges to be balanced by a tube containing a liquid of uniform density.

- As a general rule, only thick-walled tubes can be used partially filled, while thin-walled tubes for ultracentrifuges should always be completely filled to prevent them from collapsing at the very high centrifugal fields that are commonly used.

In swinging-bucket rotors, all the buckets must always be installed even though they may not all contain tubes. In the common four-place swinging buckets of low-speed or high-speed centrifuges the diametrically opposed pairs must contain tubes with liquid of the same density and volume but the material in one pair may be different to the other pair. The same is true of the six-place swinging-bucket rotors that are invariably used in ultracentrifuges, but in this case an additional symmetry is possible: two different gradients can be loaded into alternate positions, so that there will be two sets of three identical tubes at 120° to each other. The reader may occasionally encounter old style three-place swinging-bucket rotors which must naturally always contain three identical tubes.

Swinging-bucket rotors are constructed so that the rotor is only properly balanced when all buckets are in place at the correct position, i.e. the number on the buckets and their positions on the rotor must match. Those of the ultracentrifuge have each bucket and often its cap numbered, as well as the place in which it fits on the rotor. These positions must be strictly observed.

- The tube pockets of vertical rotors are sealed by some form of hex-nut which must be tightened to the recommended psi value using a torque wrench and these are only installed on pockets which contain tubes.

7.2   Use of potentially pathogenic or toxic material

Many of the buckets in swinging-bucket rotors of low-speed and high-speed centrifuges are available in specially sealed forms for use with pathogenic or toxic material. Otherwise, as long as the rotors of ultracentrifuges are sealed properly, any spillage will be contained within it. If spillage is released from the rotor in a modern centrifuge it should be contained in the sealed rotor chamber. Never use a bench-top, non-refrigerated low- or high-speed centrifuge for such material since these centrifuges are cooled by drawing air in from, and expelling air out to, the laboratory environment, thus creating aerosols of any spillages.

Using an appropriate decontaminant, the rotor should be washed out and the chamber swabbed down. For biological material, sodium dodecyl sulfate (SDS), ethylene dioxide or ethanol are permissible for the decontamination of rotors.

- For work which merits the use of a containment facility, centrifugation must be carried out within that facility. If highly pathogenic material is used, a code of practice for centrifugation work should be devised which is approved by the appropriate national health and safety authority. Consult with your local health and safety committee before carrying out such work.

7.3   Temperature control

The centrifugation of most biological material is carried out at 4°C although many cell separations are carried out at room temperature, and plasma lipoproteins usually at 16 °C. Ideally the centrifuge chamber should be pre-cooled to this temperature. In many centrifuges this can be done without the rotor being in the chamber, or while the rotor is stationary, but some older ultracentrifuges need the rotor to be spinning at low speed within the chamber. The rotor itself should also be pre-cooled, so it is best to cool rotor and chamber together. If no pre-cooling is carried out, it may take up to 1 h or longer for temperature equilibrium to occur. Rotors may alternatively be pre-cooled in a refrigerator or cold-room.

Temperature sensors in centrifuge chambers, at best, register the temperature at the surface of the rotor and at worst, the atmosphere within the chamber – not the temperature within the tube. If a rotor is not run *in vacuo*, then the higher the speed of rotation, the more likely it is that the temperature in the tube is higher than the set temperature. Each high-speed Sorvall rotor has a temperature calibration graph relating the set temperature to the tube temperature at different rotational speeds.

7.4 Operational errors and problems

Operational errors which are serious enough to cause the centrifuge to malfunction are all associated with careless or uninformed handling of the sample tubes or rotor, rather than with the actual operation of the centrifuge. The only error which may arise in the latter is setting a rotational speed greater than that permitted for the particular rotor in use. However, most modern centrifuge rotors are coded so as to prevent such a setting being accepted by the machine. Earlier models will accept and run the rotor until its speed limit is reached, then register an overspeed error and either cut the motor or continue the run at the acceptable rotor speed. There are also self-limiting rotors designed to be of sufficient mass so that the drive system is not capable of running them in excess of the maximum stipulated speed.

Failure to fill ultracentrifuge tubes adequately and/or to secure their caps (where fitted) or to seal them in accordance with the manufacturer's instructions, will cause the tubes to collapse under high centrifugal fields. Cap failures can usually be attributed to lack of routine inspection and cleaning or faulty assembly. Serious rotor imbalance can also occur if tubes collapse due to exposure to a higher than permitted RCF. Even though there are sensors to detect such imbalances and to inactivate the drive, in extreme circumstances the rotor will fail under the stress and cause serious and expensive damage.

Corrosion on rotors, particularly aluminum rotors, is caused by failure to wash thoroughly any small spillages in the rotor pockets or buckets. This can become particularly severe when heavy metal salts such as CsCl are used. Corrosion and any mechanical damage to the rotor will lead to rotor imbalance and again may eventually cause rotor failure. It is very important that all rotors are regularly checked for any sign of damage and that all rotors are inspected annually by the centrifuge manufacturer.

Under certain conditions, running at the maximum rated speed might stress the rotor excessively, thus leading to rotor failure. A rotor may therefore need to be 'derated', that is, its maximum permitted speed must be reduced. Derating is an essential practice when running solutions which will form very high-density gradients. CsCl solutions of >1.2 g ml^{-1} initially will self-generate gradients which have a very high density at the bottom of the

tube, overstressing the rotor in high centrifugal fields. In such conditions th
rotor must be derated. Vertical or near-vertical rotors in which the maximum
density CsCl is spread over the length of the tube rather than concentrate
at the bottom of the tube can withstand these stresses more effectivel
(Chapter 4) and rarely need derating. The manufacturer's literature will ind
cate the conditions that call for derating and the degree of derating needed

Modern centrifuges are designed to contain any rotor failure within th
rotor chamber. Rotor failure at high rotational speeds results in the dissip
tion of a huge amount of energy, the end result being shattering of the roto
(the buckets of swinging-bucket rotors are especially prone to this), shearin
of the drive shaft and subsequent damage to the rotor chamber itself.
thick, armored wall around the chamber ensures that major accidents, when
containment fails, are now very rare. Vibration sensors detect any imbalanc
and shut off the drive, but if any excessive vibration is noticed and the driv
is still running, switch off manually at once.

Lid-locking devices are fitted to most modern machines to prevent th
lid being opened when the rotor is spinning, but some older low-spee
machines do not have this device and the lid can be opened before the roto
stops. Never do this, and never try to increase the braking of the rotor b
applying manual pressure. This is exceedingly dangerous and, also, th
sudden change in deceleration rate will create a vortex in the centrifugatio
medium, upsetting the pellet or bands of material present.

7.5   Cleaning

Simple cleaning procedures should be routinely used for rotors and tub
caps. Washing in warm water containing a nonionic (nonalkaline) detergen
such as Teepol®, followed by rinsing in distilled water and air-drying, shoul
be the usual practice after use, and always done if spillage has occurred
Aluminum rotors are especially prone to corrosion and should never b
used with strong salt gradients. All CsCl gradients should be centrifuged i
titanium rotors.

Special attention should be paid to 'O' rings and screw-threads on rotor
and caps. Examine them for deterioration and, in the case of the 'O' rings o
rotor lids, they must be lightly smeared with vacuum grease. The 'O' rings ar
important seals divorcing the interior of the rotor and sample tubes from th
vacuum in the centrifuge chamber. Screw-threads should be free of grit o
debris which might restrict easy turning.

Adherence to these simple rules and an appreciation of the problem
that might arise will help prevent rotor failure and the consequent heav
repair bills.

8.   Sedimentation of particles in rotors

Among the centrifugation techniques described in Chapter 1, the sedimen
tation of particles into a pellet, either for the harvesting of a culture mediun
or as part of differential centrifugation, is certainly the most widely usec
technique. Although it is the most simple of centrifugation procedures, du
consideration should be given to the centrifugation conditions and roto
type. For the pelleting of particles (mammalian cells, bacteria or viruses
from a culture medium, the problem of contamination by smaller particle

is not usually a major one. The aim is to recover as much of the material as possible in as short a time as possible while using the gentlest centrifugation conditions. For differential centrifugation, however, resolution of different particle is a major consideration (Chapter 1 and Chapter 6).

8.1 Pellet formation in rotors

In *swinging-bucket rotors*, any pelleted material is symmetrically distributed in a hemispherical section at the bottom of the tube. However, during sedimentation it is only those particles in the middle of the tube which move directly to the bottom. Because the centrifugal field is radial, other particles away from the center will move first to the wall of the tube (*Figure 2.6a*); there are, however, no serious consequences of this effect for pelleting. It is only in the sector-shaped compartment of a zonal rotor that ideal sedimentation is achieved (Section 10).

In *fixed-angle rotors* the effect of the radial centrifugal field is more obvious (*Figure 2.6b*). Because the tube is held at an angle, particles migrate horizontally to the wall of the tube before moving towards the bottom of the tube. Pellets in fixed-angle rotors are naturally always asymmetrically distributed towards the outer aspect of the bottom of the tube and the effect of the horizontal centrifugal field may be observed as a trailing of the pellet on the wall of the tube away from the bottom. This effect is greater as the angle at which the tube is held to the vertical is reduced. Furthermore, decantation (or aspiration) of the supernatant from the pellet (particularly if the pellet is loosely packed) is easier the more compact the pellet is towards the bottom of the tube (i.e. in those rotors with larger tuber tube angles) – the swinging-bucket rotor and the vertical rotor could be regarded as the two limiting cases. Indeed a vertical rotor is *never* used to pellet material because the sediment would occur over the full length of the tube and unless it adheres very firmly to the tube wall, it will tend to fall off as liquid is decanted or aspirated. Thus, even though fixed-angle rotors have a shorter path-length and are therefore the more efficient (Section 8.2), the swinging-bucket

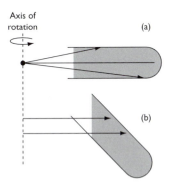

Axis of rotation

(a)

(b)

Figure 2.6

Sedimentation of particles in swinging-bucket and fixed-angle rotors. In tubes of (a) swinging-bucket rotors, particles in the center of the tube move unimpeded down the tube (axis); particles away from the axis tend to move towards the wall of the tube (the centrifugal field is radial). In tubes of (b) fixed-angle rotors, particles move first towards the outer wall of the tube.

rotor is generally preferred for the gentle pelleting of the cells. The general rule is to use the minimum RCF compatible with optimum recovery of the cells and thus reduce any compressive and hydrostatic forces on the pelleting material to a minimum. Particles can be damaged both by these forces themselves and also by the shear forces required for the resuspension of a compacted pellet.

8.2   Sedimentation path-length and the k factor

The sedimentation path-length (Section 5) of the swinging-bucket rotor is the length of the tube. In such rotors, therefore, the particles in a sample that fills the tube will experience a much lower RCF at the meniscus of the sample than at the bottom. The difference in RCF between r_{min} and r_{max} becomes more significant as the length of the tube increases. Particles at the meniscus which have the furthest to travel, either to form a pellet or to reach their buoyant density in a gradient, also experience initially the lowest RCF. The shorter the sedimentation path-length the more efficient the rotor; thus vertical rotors which have the shortest path-lengths are the most efficient for gradient centrifugation.

The k factor of a rotor takes into account its sedimentation path-length and its maximum RCF and it provides an estimate of the time (t), in hours, required to pellet a particle of known sedimentation coefficient (s), in Svedberg units, in water at 20°C, at the maximum speed of the rotor. These three parameters are related in Equation 2.3.

$$t = \frac{k}{s_{20,w}} \tag{2.3}$$

If the k factor of a rotor and the s value for a particular particle are known, then the time required to pellet the particle at the maximum speed of the rotor can be calculated.

The k factor is related to the sedimentation path-length and the angular velocity of the rotor by Equation 2.4

$$k = \frac{\ln(r_{max} - r_{min})}{\omega^2} \times \frac{10^{13}}{3600} \tag{2.4}$$

where $\omega = 0.10472 \times Q$ (r.p.m.) and r is measured in centimeters.

An alternative version of this factor, the k' factor, provides an estimate of the time required for a zone of particles to move to the bottom of a 5–20% (w/w) linear sucrose gradient at the maximum speed of the rotor. The k' factor is little used today and will not be considered further, but information on this can be found in Spragg and Steensgard (1992). Moreover, use of the k factor itself for estimating sedimentation times tends to be restricted to those particles whose sedimentation coefficient is well defined and accurately known, for example macromolecules and macromolecular complexes such as ribosomes and ribosomal subunits. Larger biological particles such as organelles and membrane vesicles are so heterogeneous that the concept is not particularly useful. It is more customary to investigate the sedimenting properties of such particles empirically. However, there is one use of the k factor which is more generally useful and that is to compare the efficiencies of different rotors.

In Equation 2.5 t_1 and k_1 are, respectively, the run time for a particular separation and the k factor of rotor 1 and t_2 and k_2 the corresponding parameters for rotor 2.

$$t_1 = \frac{k_1 t_2}{k_2} \qquad (2.5)$$

Thus a rotor with a low k factor is more efficient than one with a higher k factor and consequently will permit the more rapid separation of a particle either into a pellet or to a banding position in a gradient. *Table 2.2* lists the k factors of a few selected rotors; vertical rotors with very short sedimentation path-lengths and very high max RCFs therefore have the lowest k factors and swinging-bucket rotors with lower max RCFs have the highest k factors. Although all rotors can be assigned a k factor the parameter is principally used for ultracentrifuge rotors.

Note

Rotor manuals quote a single sedimentation path-length for a rotor, which is measured from the meniscus of a completely filled tube to the bottom of the tube. However, because of the variety of tube types and sizes which are commonly available for any one rotor, some of these may modulate the path-length and therefore the k factor. This problem is most serious with fixed-angle rotors, in which the use of open-topped tubes (which may be only partially filled) or sealed tubes may change the expected path-length quite significantly.

Many rotors can accommodate smaller volume tubes by the use of adaptors which reduce the size of the tube pocket (*Figure 2.7*). Most adaptors reduce principally the diameter of the tube and have a relatively small effect on the sedimentation path-length (*Figure 2.7b and e*), although this reduction will become more significant as the volume of the tube is reduced. Beckman g-Max® adaptors have been designed principally to reduce the path-length of swinging-bucket and fixed-angle rotors (*Figure 2.7c and f*), they also increase the r_{min} significantly, as the top of the tube is further from the axis of rotation. Traditional adaptors will also reduce the r_{max} slightly, but g-Max® adaptors have no effect on this parameter. A reduced path-length and high RCF not only makes for a more efficient separation, it is also important for the generation of gradients by the centrifugal field (self-generated gradients) which are discussed in Chapter 4.

Table 2.2. k Factors of selected Beckman–Coulter ultracentrifuge rotors

Rotor	Type[a]	Path-length (cm)	Max RCF	k factor
100 Ti	FA	3.21	802 400	15
70.1 Ti	FA	4.15	450 000	36
NVT 100	NV	1.87	750 000	8
VTi 65.1	V	1.64	402 000	13
SW60 Ti	SW	5.72	485 000	45
SW40 Ti	SW	9.21	285 000	137
TLN 120	NV	1.2	585 000	7

[a] SW, swinging-bucket; FA, fixed-angle; NV, near-vertical; V, vertical.

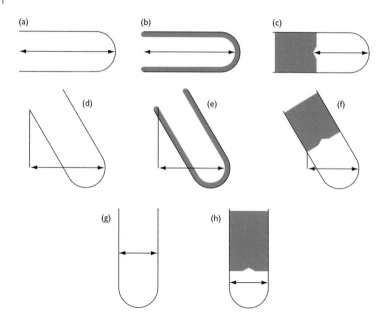

Figure 2.7

Tube adaptors. (a–c) Swinging-bucket rotor; (d–f) fixed-angle rotor; (a,d) normal; (b,e) traditional adaptor; (c,f) g-Max adaptor. Only the g-Max adaptor has a significant effect on path length. g-Max adaptors in vertical rotors (g,h) only affect the tube volume.

8.3 Hydrostatic pressure

As a guiding principle, excessive RCFs should not be used when purifying biological particles as it is well established that the hydrostatic pressures generated during centrifugation in a column of liquid can be sufficient to permeabilize membranes to gradient solutes (Sitiramam and Sarma, 1981) and to disrupt protein and nucleoprotein complexes (Marcum and Borisy, 1978 Hauge, 1971). Put simply, the magnitude of the hydrostatic pressure increases with the height of the column of liquid and the RCF. The hydrostatic pressure (P) in Nm^2 at a point in a rotating column of liquid, at a distance r (in meters) from the axis of rotation is described by Equation 2.6.

$$P = 5.48 \times 10^{-3}\, \rho\, Q^2\, (r^2 - r^2_{men}) \tag{2.6}$$

where ρ = the density of the liquid (in kg m^{-3}), Q is the rotational speed (in r.p.m.) and r_{men} = the distance (in meters) from the axis of rotation to

Table 2.3 Hydrostatic pressure (P) generated at the bottom of tubes filled with a medium $\rho = 1.10$ g ml^{-1}

Rotor	Type[a]	Tube volume (ml)	r (m)	r_{men} (m)	Q (r.p.m.)	P (kg m^{-3}
Sorvall S150AT	FA	2	0.036	0.021	150 000	116 × 10⁶
Sorvall TH660	SW	3–4	0.122	0.065	60 000	230 × 10⁶
Sorvall S120VT	V	2	0.031	0.020	120 000	49 × 10⁶
Sorvall TH641	SW	13.2	0.153	0.072	41 000	184 × 10⁶

[a]FA, fixed angle; SW, swinging-bucket; V, vertical.

the meniscus of the liquid. A few calculated examples are given in *Table 2.3*. In each case the tube is completely filled with a liquid $\rho = 1.10$ g ml^{-1}.

Although the new high-performance microultracentrifuge rotors operate at much higher Q values, it is their smaller dimensions which have the greater effect on the value of P. In a traditional swinging-bucket rotor such as the Sorvall TH-660 the hydrostatic pressure at the bottom of the tube is approximately twice that in the S-150–AT rotor operating at nearly two and a half times the r.p.m. and over four times that of the S120–VT operating at twice the r.p.m. To achieve the same hydrostatic pressure as the S150–AT, the rotational speed of the TH-660 has to be reduced to approx 42 000 r.p.m. which is equivalent to 183 000 g_{av}. To generate the same hydrostatic pressure as in the S150–AT run at top speed, the speed of larger volume swinging-bucket rotors (e.g. Sorvall TH641) must be reduced to only 33 500 r.p.m (equivalent to 140 000 g_{av}).

8.4 Selection of rotors for differential pelleting

The efficiency and/or resolution that can be achieved by differential pelleting of material (Chapters 1 and 6) is highest for rotors with a low k factor (short sedimentation path-length), thus the choice should be a fixed-angle rotor with a low angle rather than one with a larger angle or a swinging-bucket rotor. Whether the more compact pellet formation in a higher angle fixed-angle rotor is also important consideration will depend on the particular particles being pelleted.

9. Rotors for preformed density gradients

Traditionally, most density-gradient centrifugation has been carried out in swinging-bucket rotors and today this remains the most popular choice of rotor. In such rotors the walls of the tubes interfere less with the sedimenting particles than tubes in fixed-angle rotors (Section 8). Nevertheless, the effect of the radial centrifugal field in swinging-bucket rotors may be observed in the banding of particles in a gradient as a slight spreading of the band upwards at the wall of the tube. This effect is not seen if the gradients are bottom-loaded. Centrifugation times depend on the size of the particles, the viscosity of the medium and the sedimentation path-length of the rotor, which may be as long as 100 mm. So in sucrose gradients, in a rotor such as the Beckman SW28.1 or a Sorvall AH629, centrifugation times for particles such as membrane vesicles to reach isopycnic density may be at least 4–6 h (Chapter 7).

Although sedimenting particles may encounter the tube wall before they reach their banding density in fixed-angle rotors, as long as the particles do not adhere to the tube wall, there is no reason why a fixed-angle rotor should not be used. Indeed, these rotors can be used quite successfully, especially when the particle of interest is well separated from the others in the sample (Chapter 6). In the past, one of the reasons why swinging-bucket rotors were chosen for gradients was the lack of the slow, smooth acceleration facilities on centrifuges, which are needed during the reorientation of the gradient in the tube (see below). Such facilities are now widely available, making the use of shorter path-length fixed-angle rotor an attractive alternative. A fixed-angle rotor is also always capable of a higher RCF than a swinging-bucket rotor of comparable tube volume.

9.1   Vertical, near-vertical and low-angle fixed-angle rotors

High-performance rotors with short sedimentation path-lengths and lower viscosity media will speed up any gradient procedure considerably. So long as the density of the gradient at the bottom is sufficiently high to avoid the formation of a pellet, vertical rotors (with the lowest k factors) provide the most efficient way of banding particles in gradients. Vertical rotors should never be used if a pellet is formed on the wall of the tube; particles in the pellet will tend to fall back into the medium during reorientation and unloading, and thus contaminate the rest of the gradient. If some of the particles are likely to form a pellet by sedimenting completely through the gradient, then a vertical rotor should not be used and the choice should be a near-vertical or a low-angle fixed-angle rotor – or the gradient should be altered to avoid this occurrence. Vertical rotors can be particularly effective for rate-zonal separations, since any sample placed on top of a gradient achieves a very small radial thickness after reorientation (*Figure 2.8*).

In vertical and fixed-angle rotors, the plane of the gradient reorients with respect to the axis of the tube during acceleration and deceleration (*Figure 2.8*) and to minimize any mixing these phases of the centrifugation must occur smoothly and relatively slowly. Modern high-speed and ultracentrifuges have programmable acceleration and deceleration rates or at least a slow acceleration mode: the reorientation during deceleration can always be achieved without the brake. Whatever method is used to ensure a smooth reorientation of the gradient in the tube, the acceleration to and deceleration from 2000 r.p.m. should occur over approximately 5 min.

■   Because the surface area of any banded material is much higher in a vertical rotor than in a swinging-bucket rotor during centrifugation, particles which have a significant rate of diffusion ($M_r < 5 \times 10^5$) may exhibit band broadening due to this diffusion.

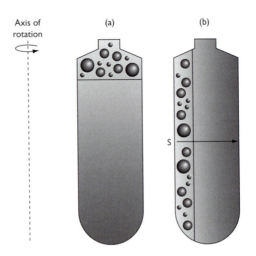

Figure 2.8

Reorientation of a gradient and sample layer in a vertical rotor during acceleration from 0 r.p.m. (a) Sample layered on top of gradient at rest. (b) After acceleration to 2000 r.p.m., gradient covers short sedimentation path length (S) and the sample occupies a narrow zone close to the axis of rotation.

Vertical, near-vertical or low-angle fixed-angle rotors are also the rotors of choice for self-generated gradients (Chapter 3).

Types of tube for gradient centrifugation

Apart from considerations of optical transparency, resistance to chemicals or sterilizing (autoclaving) procedures (Section 6), generally speaking there is no specific advantage or disadvantage of using one particular tube type for gradient centrifugation from a fractionation point of view. Choice is principally dictated by the selection of rotor type (Section 6.3), the RCF that is required (many tube types cannot be run at the maximum speed of the rotor), the degree of containment that is required and a consideration of the type of gradient harvesting that is to be carried out (Chapter 4).

10. Zonal rotors

10.1 Batch-type rotors

In zonal rotors the gradient and sample are not contained within a tube but within the body of the rotor, which is essentially a closed cylinder. The rotor which will now be briefly described is the most commonly used type of zonal rotor: it is called a batch-type rotor and operates in a routine floor-standing ultracentrifuge. These rotors have capacities of between 600 ml and 1.6 l.

The rotor comprises two half-cylinder sections which screw onto one another, an O-ring providing a water-tight seal. A central core secures a vane

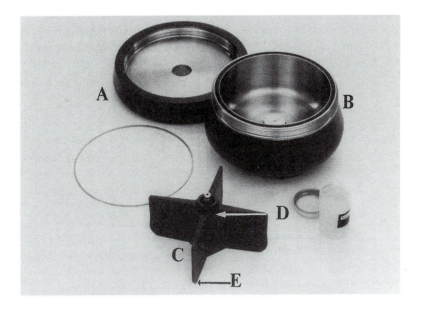

Figure 2.9

A disassembled batch-type zonal rotor (Beckman B14). The vane assembly (C) divides the hollow cylinder formed by the screwing the lid (A) on to the base of the rotor (B) into four compartments. The ports in the vane assembly allow access to the core (D) and the wall (E) of the rotor (see Figure 2.10). Reproduced from J. Graham (1992) Separations in zonal rotors. In: Preparative Centrifugation – A Practical Approach (ed. D. Rickwood). IRL Press at Oxford University Press, Oxford. With kind permission of Oxford University Press.

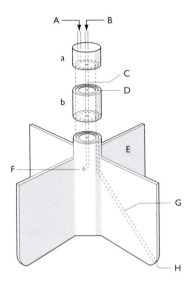

Figure 2.10

Exploded diagram of the vane and fluid seal assembly of the Beckman B14 batch-type zonal rotor. The core (F) and wall (H+G) ports on the vane assembly (F) terminate in a central channel (C) and an annulus (D) respectively, which continue upwards through the lower rotating part of the fluid seal (b). The upper (static) part of the fluid seal (a) contains the same central channel and annulus. When the rotor is spinning at 2000 r.p.m. in the open centrifuge chamber, a tray fitted into the top of the chamber mechanically restrains the static part (a) from rotating and also applies pressure at the polished apposed faces of the two parts of the fluid seal. The annulus and central channel of the static seal emerge as two tubes (A and B, respectively); thus, the rotor can be loaded with gradient and sample while spinning at low speed. After loading, the static seal is removed and the rotor capped allowing the chamber to be closed and the rotor accelerated for the separation phase. The rotor is decelerated to 2000 rpm; the chamber opened and the static seal reinstated, allowing the gradient to be unloaded. Reproduced from J. Graham (1992) Separations in zonal rotors. In: Preparative Centrifugation – A Practical Approach (ed. D. Rickwood). IRL Press at Oxford University Press, Oxford. With kind permission of Oxford University Press.

(septa) assembly which fits over the core and divides the enclosed space into four sectors (*Figure 2.9*). The core also contains two channels: an annulus, which is continuous with a channel in each of the vanes and thus allows access to the edge of the rotor, and a central channel, which exits at the surface of the core. This rotor is able to spin at about 2000 r.p.m. with the centrifuge chamber door open; in this mode a 'feed head' or 'fluid seal' is positioned on top of the rotating core (*Figure 2.10*). The lower half of the fluid seal is allowed to rotate with the rotor, within a bearing housing, while the top half is constrained from rotation mechanically. As both halves of the fluid seal contain a central core and an annulus to match those in the core of the rotor, it is possible to pump fluid either to the edge of the spinning rotor or to its core. In this way, once the rotor has been filled with gradient (via the annular channel) from the edge (low-density end first), the sample is applied to the gradient through the central channel and subsequently the radial position of the sample band and the gradient volume can be manipulated by pumping either low-density liquid to the core or high-density liquid to the edge.

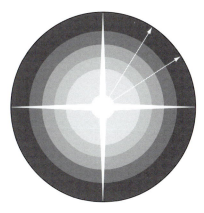

Figure 2.11

Ideal sedimentation in a zonal rotor. The gradient is contained within sector-shaped compartments; the sedimenting particles never encounter a radial surface (compare Figure 2.6).

Once the gradient and sample have been pumped into the spinning rotor, the fluid seal is removed, the rotor capped off and the chamber door closed. The rotor is then accelerated to its running speed and operated like any other rotor. After the separation has occurred the rotor is decelerated back to 2000 r.p.m. and the fluid seal reinstated. Unloading the rotor is normally achieved by pumping dense unloading medium to the edge of the rotor and thus displacing the gradient (low-density end first) via the core. The effluent is customarily monitored by passing it through the flow cell of a recording spectrophotometer and collected in a fraction collector. For more operational detail, see Graham (1992).

Of all the rotor types, this is the only one which provides the conditions for optimal resolution of biological particles. *Figure 2.11* is a diagrammatic representation of a horizontal cross-section through the spinning rotor, which shows the cylindrical blocks of a discontinuous gradient and the arrows show lines of radial centrifugal force along which particles sediment. This is ideal sedimentation in a sector-shaped compartment; particles never collide with a surface unless they reach the wall of the rotor, which is never allowed to happen. Because the rotors are loaded and unloaded dynamically (i.e. while the rotor is spinning), gradient disturbances that may occur during acceleration or deceleration to rest and handling of rotors cannot occur.

Unloading the rotor from the core by displacement with a dense medium is also ideal, the zonal effluent being collected in a progressively tapering conical section.

For rate-zonal separations in particular, zonal rotors provide the highest resolution. By moving the sample away from the core of the rotor with a lower density overlay, the sample occupies an exponentially decreasing radial distance. A sample of 35 ml, for example, can easily occupy a radial thickness of less than 3 mm. To achieve this in a large volume swinging-bucket rotor (e.g. a Beckman SW28) would require at least 24 tubes. Batch-type zonal rotors are therefore very successfully used for fractionating ribosomal subunits and polysomes (Graham, 1992). Indeed these are two important applications of zonal rotors, but the most widely used application is probably the harvesting and purification of virus from up to 1.5 l of culture fluid (Graham, 1992).

There are variants (mainly for high-speed centrifuges) which allow loading and/or unloading while the rotor is stationary. Although such rotors can dispense with the need for a fluid seal, the advantages of dynamic loading and unloading are of course lost. Others have modified cores and vanes which allow collection of the gradient from the edge or the use of just a small volume of the rotor space close to the edge of the rotor. In the 1960s and 1970s, these rotors attained a degree of popularity which has waned considerably since that time. There will always be an occasional requirement for large-scale isolation and these rotors are the rotors of choice, but their use requires considerable expertise and great care in handling and maintaining the fluid seal.

10.2 Continuous-flow zonal rotors

The overall design of these rotors is the same as for the batch type-rotors, that is, they allow the gradient to be loaded and unloaded while the rotor is spinning at a low speed and there are variants which permit these operations to be carried out while the rotor is stationary. The one significant difference, however, is that the fluid lines within the core allow the sample to be

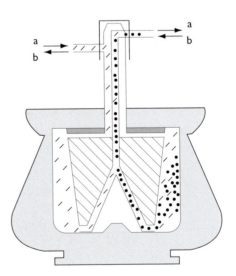

Figure 2.12

A continuous-flow zonal rotor. Not only is the rotor loaded with gradient and unloaded while spinning at 2000 r.p.m., a specially constructed chamber lid allows the complete fluid seal to be in place also during the separation phase at up to 40 000 r.p.m. The channels within the vane assembly are modified so that while the rotor is spinning, virus-containing fluid, for example, can be pumped into the rotor using path (b). When the fluid reaches the bottom of the vane, because it is less dense than the top of the gradient already in the rotor (introduced previously at 2000 r.p.m. through path a), it flows up over the core of the rotor, allowing the viral particles to sediment out into the gradient. From J. Graham (1992) Separations in zonal rotors. In: Preparative Centrifugation – A Practical Approach (ed. D. Rickwood). IRL Press at Oxford University Press, Oxford. With kind permission of Oxford University Press.

pumped to the bottom of the core in a low-density medium which flows up over the core surface while the rotor is running at the separation speed (30 000–40 000 r.p.m. in ultracentrifuges). During the flow of the sample over the core surface, the biological particles sediment out into the gradient and the particle-free liquid emerges from the top of the core (*Figure 2.12*). In ultracentrifuges this requires a more complex fluid seal to be in place during the entire operation within the evacuated centrifuge chamber. It is less of a problem for high-speed centrifuges.

In ultracentrifuges, continuous-flow zonal rotors are used principally for the harvesting of virus from very large volumes (10–20 l) of culture fluid, while those for high-speed rotors can be used for similar volumes of bacterial cultures. For more information on their mode of use and specific protocols, see Graham (1992).

11. The analytical ultracentrifuge

A useful description of the hardware and operation of the analytical ultracentrifuge for the determination of the mass and shape of macromolecules is beyond the remit of this text. Only a few brief comments about one of its principal modes of operation will be made.

The samples under investigation are contained within wedge-shaped optically transparent cells which are mounted within the rotor (*Figure 2.13*). As with all centrifugal systems the macromolecules can be analyzed by sedimentation velocity or sedimentation equilibrium.

In *moving boundary analysis* the cell is initially filled (except for a small air gap at the top of the cell) with a homogenous solution of a protein solution

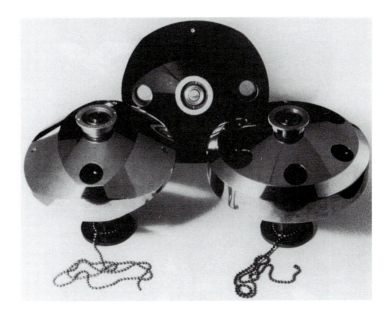

Figure 2.13

A selection of analytical rotors showing the apertures for accommodating the cell assemblies. Reproduced from R. Eason (1984) Analytical ultracentrifugation. In: Centrifugation – A Practical Approach *(ed. D. Rickwood). IRL Press at Oxford University Press, Oxford. With kind permission of R. Eason and Oxford University Press.*

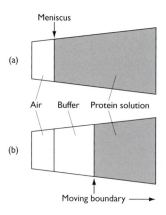

Meniscus

(a)

Air   Buffer   Protein solution

(b)

Moving boundary ⟶

Figure 2.14

Moving boundary analysis. (a) At time zero the cell is filled with the protein solution, leaving a small air gap. (b) When the protein molecules sediment, a protein-free buffer phase is formed. The rate of movement of the boundary between the protein-free buffer and the increasingly concentrated protein solution is measured optically. Reproduced from R. Eason (1984) Analytical ultracentrifugation. In: Centrifugation – A Practical Approach *(ed. D. Rickwood). IRL Press at Oxford University Press, Oxford. With kind permission of R. Eason and Oxford University Press.*

in a suitable buffer. During centrifugation the protein molecules sediment at a rate which depends on their size and shape, thus a moving boundary is formed within the cell between the increasing protein-free buffer solution on top and the protein solution below (*Figure 2.14*). Because the wall of the cell is optically transparent, the movement of the boundary can be monitored. If the macromolecules have a significant and characteristic absorbance at a particular wavelength, then either photographs may be taken using a UV source of fixed wavelength, or a photoelectric scanner-monochromator can be used. Alternatively, the progress of the moving boundary may be monitored by the changes in refractive index which occur in the cell using either Schlieren or Rayleigh optics. The absorbance or refractive index changes in the test cell are compared with a reference cell in the rotor containing only buffer and the progress of the boundary recorded continuously.

Sedimentation velocities of proteins can also be determined using a system not unlike that described in Chapter 8, in which the sample is applied as a narrow zone upon either a pre-formed or self-generated gradient.

For a review of the use of these and other strategies, see Eason (1984).

References

Eason, R. (1984) Analytical ultracentrifugation. In: *Centrifugation – A Practical Approach*, 2nd edn (ed. D. Rickwood). IRL Press at Oxford University Press, Oxford, pp. 251–286.

Graham, J.M. (1992) Separations in zonal rotors. In: *Preparative Centrifugation – A Practical Approach* (ed. D. Rickwood). IRL Press at Oxford University Press, Oxford, pp. 219–249.

Hauge, J.G. (1971) Pressure-induced dissociation of ribosomes during centrifugation. *FEBS Lett.* **17**: 168–172.

Marcum, J.M. and Borisy, G.G. (1978) Sedimentation velocity analyses of the effect of hydrostatic pressure on the 30S microtubule protein oligomer. *J. Biol. Chem.* **253**: 2852–2857.

Rickwood, D. (1992a) Appendix 2, Specifications of ultracentrifuge rotors. In: *Preparative Centrifugation – A Practical Approach* (ed. D. Rickwood). IRL Press at Oxford University Press, Oxford, pp. 355–365.

Rickwood, D. (1992b) Appendix 1, Chemical resistance chart for tubes, adapters and rotor materials. In: *Preparative Centrifugation – A Practical Approach* (ed. D. Rickwood). IRL Press at Oxford University Press, Oxford, pp. 351–353.

Sitiramam, V. and Sarma, M.J.K. (1981) Gravitational field enhances permeability of biological membranes to sucrose: an experimental refutation of sucrose-space hypothesis. *Proc. Natl Acad. Sci. USA* **78**: 3441–3445.

Spragg, S.P. and Steensgard, J. (1992) Theoretical aspects of practical centrifugation. In: *Preparative Centrifugation – A Practical Approach* (ed. D. Rickwood). IRL Press at Oxford University Press, Oxford, pp. 1–42.

Chapter 3

Gradient media

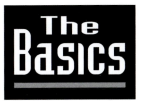

This chapter confines itself to a discussion of the general requirements of gradient media, a description of their physicochemical properties, how suitable gradient solutions are produced, how the density of their solutions is measured and how the media may affect subsequent analytical techniques. Their suitability to the isolation of specific types of biological particle is covered in the relevant chapters (Chapters 5–8).

1. Choosing a suitable density-gradient medium

1.1 Effect on biological particles

The objective of density-gradient centrifugation is to separate particles, either on the basis of their buoyant (also called banding, equilibrium or isopycnic) density or their rate or velocity of sedimentation in a medium which causes the least potential damage to the particles of interest. Sometimes the aim (preparative) is to purify a single specific type of particle in order to determine its structure and function; sometimes the aim (analytical) is to obtain optimum separation of a range of different particles in order to determine the localization or distribution of a particular component or function. Investigations of complex cellular processes such as secretion and endocytosis often involve the use of density gradients to assess the progress of macromolecules through a series of membrane compartments (Chapter 7).

Some of the first differential and density-gradient centrifugation techniques that were developed in the early 1950s were for the purification of cell organelles. As buffered 0.25 M sucrose became the homogenization medium of choice for mammalian tissues, it was a natural extension to use sucrose as the medium for constructing density gradients. Because sucrose was cheap and relatively inert, it achieved wide acceptance as a gradient medium.

In choosing a solute as a gradient medium, it must naturally satisfy the prime need of being able to form solutions of a wide range of densities. There are additionally two other important physical parameters which influence the suitability of a solute as a gradient medium: its viscosity and its osmolality. Viscosity affects the rate at which a particle sediments through the medium (Section 2); high viscosity leads to long centrifugation times. The osmolality affects the hydration of the particles passing through the gradient. High osmolality solutions not only remove water from the enclosed space of osmotically active particles – and that includes most membrane-bound particles – they also remove water molecules bound to macromolecules (such as DNA) and macromolecular complexes (such as ribonucleoproteins and viruses). Although the osmotic effect may be reversible when the particle has been separated and transferred back to an isoosmotic environment, it is clearly a possible source of structural and functional change which is best avoided. Loss of water from a biological particle will increase its density and, in the case of membrane-bound organelles markedly reduce its size, in this way the rate at which a particle sediments and its buoyant density are going to be continuously modified as it passes through a gradient of increasing osmolality.

The osmolality of most mammalian fluids, both intracellular and extracellular, is 290–300 mOsm. This is the osmolality of the common media for suspending mammalian particles: 0.85–0.9% (w/v) NaCl (or other balanced salt solutions) and 0.25 M sucrose. It should be pointed out, however, that the subcellular particles of other systems (plant, yeast, etc.) are routinely isolated in media of slightly higher osmotic activity (e.g. 0.3–0.8 M sorbitol).

Consideration of the possible effect of osmolality on the biological particles is part of a more general aim of any protocol, which must be to conserve the form and function of the particle as closely as possible to that of its natural state. While it must always be borne in mind that the very separation of particles from their natural environment is likely to alter their structure and function to a lesser or greater degree, every effort must be made to minimize such changes by ensuring that the gradient medium in which the biological particles are suspended is compatible with the particles. Thus, just as important as the physicochemical parameters of a gradient medium are its biological properties.

The medium should obviously not be toxic or injurious to the particles. Cells are particularly stringent in their requirements for a suitable solute and many of the media which are tolerated by subcellular particles and macromolecules are totally unsuited to cells. The gradient solute should not be absorbed on to the surface of the particles, nor should it affect ionic or nonionic interactions between groups on macromolecules. In the case of cells, organelles and membrane vesicles, the solute should not cross the limiting membrane.

Table 3.1 summarizes the general usage of gradient media for the major biological particle types.

1.2   Other considerations

Consideration should also be given to the possible interference between the gradient medium and any processing or analytical techniques subsequent to the separation. Thus it should be easy to remove from the particles if required. There is evidence that certain enzymes are sensitive to particular media and some standard chemical measurements cannot be carried out in the presence of some media (or some media above a certain concentration). See Section 4.1 for more information.

Finally, the availability of particular centrifugation hardware may also influence the choice of medium since it may be possible to use a method in which a self-generated gradient is used rather than a pre-formed one. Only a few of the gradient media are able to form self-generated gradients and recent advances in centrifuge and rotor technology may permit separations in such gradients to take place in much reduced times (Chapter 4).

Table 3.1. Density-gradient media and their principal uses

Gradient medium type	Principal uses and comments
Polyhydric alcohols	
Sucrose	Organelles, membrane vesicles, viruses, proteins, ribosomes, polysomes
Glycerol	Mammalian cells (infrequent), proteins
Sorbitol	Nonmammalian subcellular particles
Polysaccharides	
Ficoll®, polysucrose and dextrans	Mammalian cells (sometimes in combination with iodinated density gradient media), mammalian subcellular particles (infrequent).
Inorganic salts	
CsCl	DNA, viruses, proteins
Cs_2SO_4	DNA and RNA
KBr	Plasma lipoproteins
Iodinated gradient media	
Diatrizoate	Mainly as a component of commercial lymphocyte isolation media
Nycodenz®	Mammalian cells, organelles, membrane vesicles, viruses
Iodixanol	Mammalian cells, organelles, membrane vesicles, viruses, plasma lipoproteins, proteins, DNA
Colloidal silica media	
Percoll®	Mammalian cells, organelles, membrane vesicles (infrequent)

1.3 Types of gradient media

Over the last 30 years or more, a number of different compounds (both inorganic and organic) have been investigated as density-gradient media in order to enhance the separation process, to overcome the problems of osmolality and viscosity, to improve the retention of the biological activity of the particles and, in particular, to separate particles for which sucrose is unsuitable. There are now five main classes of density gradient medium: (i) polyhydric alcohols, (ii) polysaccharides, (iii) inorganic salts, (iv) iodinated compounds based on metrizoic acid and (v) colloidal silica. Examples of these classes and their principal uses are given in *Table 3.1*. The chemical nature of the iodinated density gradient media and colloidal silica may be unfamiliar to the reader and these will now be briefly described.

Metrizamide and Nycodenz®

The iodinated media, derived from metrizoic acid, were originally developed for use as X-ray contrast media (Rickwood, 1984). Sodium metrizoate and a closely related compound, diatrizoate (*Figure 3.1*), form ionic solutions in water and they are relatively little used today as general-purpose density-gradient media (but see *Table 3.1*).

Further development of the X-ray contrast media resulted in the production of a series of nonionic, iodinated media, which were both clinically more acceptable and more useful as density-gradient media. The first of these (metrizamide) was available in the early 1970s; in this molecule the

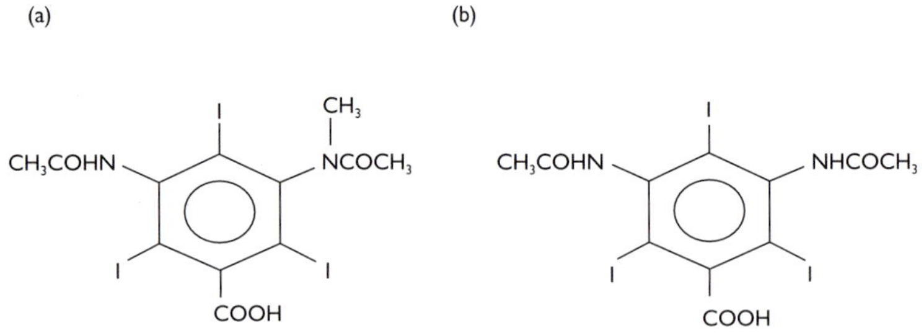

(a)   (b)

Figure 3.1

Molecular structure of metrizoic acid (a) and diatrizoic acid (b).

free COOH group of metrizoic acid was linked to glucosamine (*Figure 3.2a*). In the early 1980s Nycodenz® was introduced; it is a trademark name for iohexol whose systematic name is 5-(N-2,3–dihydroxypropylacetamido)-2,4,6–triiodo-N,N′-bis(2,3-dihydroxypropyl) isophthalamide. It has a molecular weight of 821 (*Figure 3.2b*). The carboxyl group of metrizoic acid is linked to the amine group of 3-amino-1,2-propanediol rather than to glucosamine. The heavily hydroxylated side-chains of the Nycodenz® molecule make it highly hydrophilic and more readily water soluble than metrizamide.

Iodixanol

In the early 1990s iodixanol was developed as an X-ray contrast medium; it is essentially a dimer of Nycodenz® and thus has almost twice its molecular mass (*Figure 3.3*). Its systematic chemical name is 5,5′-[(2-hydroxy-1-3-propanediyl)-bis(acetylamino)]bis[N,N′bis(2,3-dihydroxypropyl)-2,4,6-triiodo-1,3-benzenecarboxamide]. Iodixanol is available commercially as a 60% (w/v) solution in water called OptiPrep™.

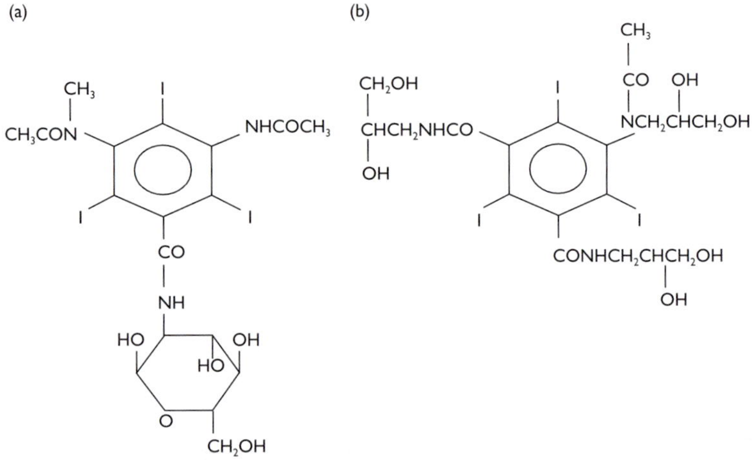

(a)   (b)

Figure 3.2

Molecular structure of metrizamide (a) and Nycodenz® (b).

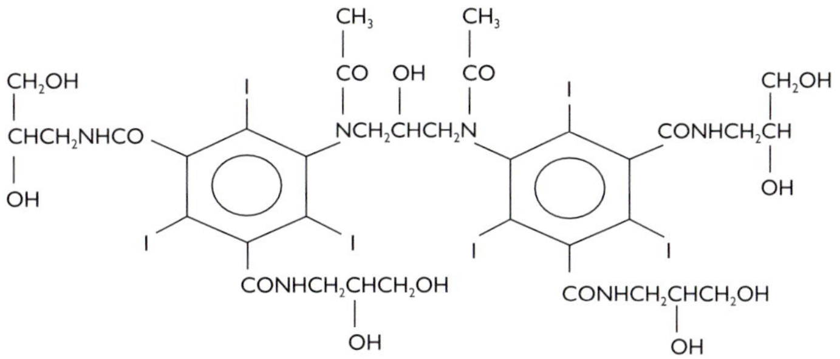
CH3
CH3
CO OH CO
CH2OH
NCH2CHCH2N
CH2OH
CHCH2NHCO
CONHCH2CH
OH
OH
I
I
I
I
I
I
CONHCH2CHCH2OH
OH
CONHCH2CHCH2OH
OH

Figure 3.3

Molecular structure of iodixanol.

Colloidal silica

Colloidal silica media are, as the name implies, colloidal suspensions of silica particles and not true solutions. They were first recognized as possible density-gradient media in the early 1960s. Unmodified silica particles, however, were found to be toxic to cells and unstable in salt solutions. Stability was increased by coating the particles with polymers such as dextran, polyethylene glycol (PEG) or polyvinylpyrrolidone (PVP), which also decreased their toxicity (Pertoft *et al.*, 1977; 1978). The most widely known and used of the colloidal media is that marketed under the name of Percoll®. Percoll® is a colloidal suspension of PVP-coated silica particles of 15–30 nm diameter with a density of 1.130 g ml^{-1}. Percoll® also contains a small amount of free PVP, to which some cells are very sensitive; in the commercial medium Redigrad® the colloidal silica is stabilized by silane rather than PVP. Some other colloidal silica media are discussed by Rickwood (1984).

2. Physicochemical characteristics of gradient media

Figures 3.4, 3.5 and *3.6* compare respectively the density, osmolality and viscosity of a number of different types of gradient medium; in each figure the parameter is plotted against concentration of gradient medium in % (w/v) and they should be referred to in the following descriptions of the media.

2.1 Polyhydric alcohols

Sucrose is by far the most widely used of any gradient medium and solutions can be prepared with densities up to 1.39 g ml^{-1}. It is freely soluble in water, although at the highest concentrations (approximately 67%, w/w) the extreme viscosity makes dissolution difficult and slow. Solutions of sucrose are hyperosmotic at concentrations above 9.0% (w/v); this is equivalent to a density of approximately 1.03 g ml^{-1}. The banding of any particles under isoosmotic conditions is therefore not possible in sucrose. All osmotically active particles will therefore continuously lose water and increase their density as they move through a sucrose gradient. The high viscosity of sucrose solutions also leads to slow sedimentation velocities and long centrifugation times (often more than 6 h). Viscosity is highly temperature-

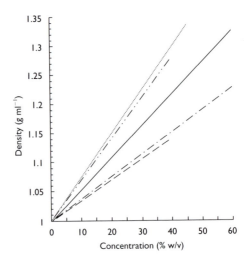

Figure 3.4

Density vs. concentration of solutions of different gradient media. CsCl (······), Percoll® (— ··), iodixanol (——), sucrose (— ·), Ficoll (– –). Note that the density curve of Nycodenz® (not shown) is virtually identical to that of iodixanol.

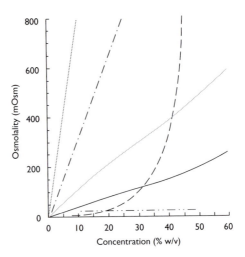

Figure 3.5

Osmolality vs. concentration of solutions of different gradient media. Nycodenz® (——), for other line identities see Figure 3.4.

dependent (*Table 3.2*) and if the temperature of gradients is not carefully controlled (see Chapter 2), then rates of sedimentation of particles in sucrose and other media will vary from run to run.

■   The viscosity of sucrose gradients can be reduced by substituting D_2O for H_2O (the former has a density of 1.11 g ml^{-1}, against 0.998 g ml^{-1} for water).

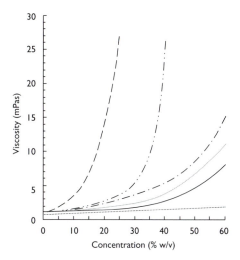

Figure 3.6

Viscosity vs. concentration of solutions of different gradient media. For line identities see Figures 3.4 and 3.5.

2.2   Polysaccharides

Because of the high osmolality of solutions of sucrose and other polyhydric alcohols, the use of high molecular mass polysaccharides, such as the naturally occurring dextrans and the synthetic Ficoll® (polysucrose), were introduced as density-gradient media. For any given concentration, solutions of polysaccharides (compared to those of sucrose) have a rather similar density, but as a consequence of their high molecular mass, a much lower osmolality. However, it is only at relatively low concentrations (below 25%) that the osmolality of Ficoll® is very low (less than 50 mOsm). As the concentration rises above 25% the osmolality increases sharply as the number of free water molecules in the solution declines. Solutions of these polysaccharides (below 30%) successfully overcome the osmolality problem displayed by sucrose; on the other hand, the viscosity of the solutions is much higher leading to much longer centrifugation times. Polysaccharides are rarely used above 30% (w/v) which is equivalent to a density of approximately 1.10 g ml^{-1}, moreover the preparation of solutions is difficult and time-consuming.

Table 3.2. Effect of temperature on the viscosity of sucrose solutions

%	Viscosity (centipoises) at °C				
(w/w)	0	5	10	15	20
20	3.77	3.14	2.64	2.55	1.95
30	6.67	5.42	4.48	3.76	3.19
40	14.58	11.45	9.16	7.46	6.16
50	44.74	33.16	25.17	19.52	15.42

2.3   Solutions of heavy metal salts

Among the salts of the various heavy metals, CsCl and Cs_2SO_4 are probably the most widely used as centrifugation media. Solutions with densities of up to 1.9 and 2.01 g ml^{-1} respectively, can be prepared and although the viscosity of these solutions is very low, they are highly hyperosmotic. The available 'free' water molecules in a solution, that is, water molecules not bound to the solute, is an important factor and defines the term 'water activity' of a solution: in one with a low water activity there are few free water molecules in one with a high water activity there are many. The importance of the water activity of a solution used as a density-gradient medium is seen in the effect it has upon the degree of hydration of biological particles exposed to it. In solutions of low water activity (e.g. high concentrations of CsCl), biological particles, such as DNA, tend to become partially dehydrated, while in solutions of high activity they will be closer to the fully hydrated state. The buoyant density of DNA in CsCl gradients is observed to be about 1.6–1.7 g ml^{-1}, while in solutions with higher water activities, such as those of Nycodenz or iodixanol it bands at a density of 1.11–1.12 g ml^{-1}.

2.4   Other inorganic salts

The physicochemical properties of the higher halides of sodium and potassium are not unlike those of the heavy metal salts. Alkali metal salts such as NaI and KI have be used for the isopycnic banding of nucleic acids. KI gradients in particular seem to avoid the problem of RNA aggregation (Rickwood 1992). KBr is widely used for the fractionation of human plasma lipoproteins (Chapter 8), but because of the nature of lipoproteins, the water activity of the medium has relatively little effect on their density although the particularly high ionic strength of the media used to isolate high-density lipoprotein (HDL) may have an effect on the hydration of its proteins.

2.5   Iodinated density-gradient media

Both metrizamide and Nycodenz® can provide solutions (up to approximately 1.43 g ml^{-1}) but for most purposes densities above approximately 1.30 g ml^{-1} are not required. Moreover the osmolality of these solutions are much lower than those of sucrose and inorganic salts of the same density (*Figure 3.5*). Particles in these media are therefore much more highly hydrated than in solutions of sucrose or inorganic salts and consequently their densities are generally much lower (see Chapters 6–8). Solutions of Nycodenz® are hyperosmotic only above approximately 1.155 g ml^{-1} and even at higher densities, the osmolality is much lower than that of sucrose or salts. Metrizamide solutions become hyperosmotic above approximately 1.185 g ml^{-1}. Only solutions of inorganic salts have lower viscosities than those of Nycodenz® or metrizamide (*Figure 3.6*) and particles therefore sediment very rapidly in these media. In terms of their ability to separate biological particles, the two compounds are very similar; a separation technique describing the use of one is likely to be easily adapted to the other.

   The chemical and physical properties of iodixanol are similar to those of Nycodenz®, but because it has twice the molecular mass of Nycodenz®, solutions of iodixanol have about half the osmotic activity (*Figure 3.5*). Consequently solutions of this compound can be made isoosmotic at all useful densities (Section 3.3) and all biological particles can be isolated under isoosmotic conditions. The viscosity of its solutions is slightly higher than those of Nycodenz® or metrizamide. It has the same wide spectrum of applications as the other two nonionic media.

2.6 Percoll®

Being a colloidal suspension, Percoll® itself has essentially no osmotic activity and can therefore provide gradient solutions of any osmolality that is required by addition of a suitable solute. The viscosity of Percoll solutions is slightly higher than those of inorganic salts or the iodinated media (*Figure 3.6*) and increases markedly above 30% (w/v). Densities greater than 1.130 g ml^{-1} can only be formed during self-generated gradient formation (Chapter 4).

3. Preparing solutions of gradient media

3.1 General strategies

It is common practice to prepared stock-buffered solutions of gradient media at high concentration which can be subsequently further diluted with buffer to produce solutions of the appropriate density (Section 3.3). Stocks of inorganic salts can be kept almost indefinitely at 4°C; stocks of polyhydric alcohols and polysaccharides are very prone to microbial contamination, even at very high concentrations and when kept at 4°C. Storage of these solutions at −20°C is a possibility but not really very convenient.

It may often be desirable to perform a gradient separation under sterile conditions and autoclaving can provide some unexpected problems. The silica particle suspension of Percoll® is destabilized during autoclaving in the presence of salts or sucrose; therefore all Percoll® diluents must be autoclaved separately. Of the iodinated density gradient media, only metrizamide cannot be autoclaved – neither can sucrose or polysaccharide solutions.

Iodixanol is only available commercially as OptiPrep™ (a 60% w/v solution). Nycodenz® is also available as a solution at an identical concentration (NycoPrep™ Universal) but also as a powder. Solutions from a powder are best produced by adding the powder to water while stirring at approximately 80°.

Dissolution of polysaccharides is facilitated by adding small volumes of water to the powder and stirring after each addition to produce a thick translucent paste before diluting to the required volume. If water is added directly to the powder it tends to form a large aggregated mass.

3.2 Measurement of density

The density of gradient solutions and gradient fractions of all media can be assessed either by pycnometry or by refractometry. Pycnometry involves the weighing of a known volume of solution using a density bottle (an approximate estimate for solutions of low viscosity can be obtained by weighing a volume dispensed from a calibrated automatic pipette). This is not convenient for the measurement of large numbers of fractions. Refractometry is by far the most widely used method; it uses only about 25 μl of sample and a simple formula (Equation 3.1) allows quick and accurate calculation of the density from the refractive index. The density values in *Table 3.5*, for example, were calculated using $A = 3.466$ and $B = 3.632$.

$$\rho = A\eta - B. \tag{3.1}$$

The values of these constants (A and B) which vary with the gradient solute and the osmotic balancer can be easily computed from a graph of ρ versus η as all of the lines are described by $y = mx + c$. The density of any solution produced by dilution of a working solution with a diluent can deduced from Equation 3.2.

$$D = \frac{Vd + V_1 d_1}{V + V_1} \tag{3.2}$$

D = Required density; V = volume of working (or stock) solution; d = density of working (or stock) solution; V_1 = volume of diluent; d_1 = density of diluent.

The density and refractive index of some commonly used gradient media and their diluents are given in *Table 3.3*.

Although Percoll® is not a true solution and the figures provided by the refractometer are not a true refractive index, they can nevertheless be used to determine the density of Percoll® solutions following calibration with solutions of known density. Alternatively, colored density marker beads are available which can provide an indication of the density profile of Percoll® gradients.

3.3   Osmotic balancers and isoosmotic gradients

Sucrose and inorganic salts

Density gradients of sucrose (and other polyhydric alcohols) and inorganic salts must also be gradients of viscosity and osmolality and there is no way in which either of these parameters can be modulated independently. Isoosmotic solutions of these solutes are equivalent to concentrations (approximately 0.25 M sucrose and 0.145 M NaCl) well below those used for gradients (*Figure 3.5*). Thus, any gradient even at its lowest density will be hyperosmotic.

Polysaccharides

The nature of the osmolality curve of polysaccharides makes it impossible to use these to prepare isoosmotic gradients above a density of approximately 1.08 g ml^{-1} (*Figures 3.4* and *3.5*). For mammalian cell work, concentration

Table 3.3. Density (ρ) and refractive index (η) of some commonly used solutions

Solution	ρ (g ml^{-1})	η
0.25 M sucrose in 10 mM Tris/Hepes/Tricine	1.03	1.3450
0.85% saline in 10 mM Hepes	1.005	1.3350
2.5 M sucrose	1.3163	1.4532
OptiPrep™ (60% w/v) iodixanol	1.32	1.4287
60% (w/v) Nycodenz®	1.319	1.4318
Percoll®	1.13	1.3540
4 M CsCl	1.497	1.3807

of below 25% (w/v) are simply prepared by dissolving the solute in a routine balanced salt or saline solution; the density solutions will be very close to isoosmotic.

Iodinated density gradient media

A 60% (w/v) Nycodenz®, 10 mM Tris–HCl, pH 7.4 solution has an osmolality of approximately 590 mOsm and if diluted with its buffer, the solutions will be increasingly hyperosmotic above approximately 30% Nycodenz® and increasingly hypoosmotic below this value (*Figure 3.5*). On the other hand, if an approximately isoosmotic solution of 30% (w/v) Nycodenz® solution is diluted with a solution which is also isoosmotic (an osmotic balancer) then all the dilutions will also be isoosmotic. For mammalian organelles, the osmotic balancer will be 0.25 M sucrose, 10 mM Tris–HCl, pH 7.4 (*Table 3.4*); for mammalian cells it would be a balanced salt solution or buffered saline (*Table 3.5*).

The easiest medium to handle for the preparation of isoosmotic solutions at all densities is OptiPrep™ (compare with the handling of Percoll® below). OptiPrep™, being a 60% (w/v) solution of iodixanol in water, has an osmolality of approximately 170 mOsm. This is lower than might be expected when compared with Nycodenz®, for although iodixanol is double the molecular mass of Nycodenz®, the osmolality of a 60% (w/v) solution is less than a third of that of Nycodenz®. This is because at high concentrations the molecule tends to associate into oligomers. When OptiPrep™ is diluted with a buffer, however, these oligomers dissociate so that the osmolality approaches the expected value. As a result, the normal way of preparing isoosmotic density solutions of iodixanol is to prepare first a working solution (or working stock) of 40% or 50% iodixanol which contains the required buffer and additives and then dilute this with the regular cell suspension medium or homogenization medium.

Table 3.4. Properties of Nycodenz®–sucrose solutions[a]

% Nycodenz (w/v)	η	ρ (g ml⁻¹)
0.00	1.3450	1.030
2.50	1.3481	1.041
5.00	1.3512	1.052
7.50	1.3544	1.062
10.00	1.3575	1.073
12.50	1.3606	1.084
15.00	1.3637	1.095
17.50	1.3668	1.105
20.00	1.3699	1.116
22.50	1.3731	1.127
25.00	1.3762	1.138
27.50	1.3793	1.148
30.00	1.3824	1.159

[a] 30% Nycodenz , 10 mM Tris–HCl, pH 7.4 is diluted with 0.25 M sucrose, 10 mM Tris–HCl, pH 7.4.
η, refractive index; ρ, density. The osmolality of the gradient solutions is in the range 290–315 mOsm.

Table 3.5. Properties of Nycodenz®–saline solutions[a]

% Nycodenz (w/v)	η	ρ (g ml⁻¹)
0.00	1.3350	1.005
2.50	1.3390	1.018
5.00	1.3429	1.031
7.50	1.3469	1.044
10.00	1.3508	1.056
12.50	1.3548	1.069
15.00	1.3587	1.082
17.50	1.3627	1.095
20.00	1.3666	1.108
22.50	1.3706	1.120
25.00	1.3745	1.133
27.50	1.3785	1.146
30.00	1.3824	1.159

[a] 30% Nycodenz, 10 mM Tricine–NaOH, pH 7.4 is diluted with 0.85% NaCl, 10 mM Tricine–NaOH, pH 7.4.
η, refractive index; ρ, density. The osmolality of the gradient solutions is in the range 285–305 mOsm.

■ Thus for organelles if the homogenization medium (HM) contains 0.25 M sucrose, 1 mM EDTA, 10 mM Tris–HCl, pH 7.4; a working solution containing 50% iodixanol is prepared from 5 volumes of Optiprep™ and 1 volume of 0.25 M sucrose, 6 mM EDTA, 60 mM Tris–HCl, pH 7.4. This is further diluted with the HM (*Table 3.6*). The buffer and EDTA concentrations in the density solutions will be constant.

■ For mammalian cells, a 40% iodixanol working solution is prepared from 4 volumes of OptiPrep™ and 2 volumes of 0.85% NaCl, 30 mM Tricine–NaOH, pH 7.4. This is further diluted with 0.85% NaCl, 10 mM Tricine–NaOH, pH 7.4 (*Table 3.7*).

If density solutions are simply prepared by dilution of OptiPrep' with the routine HM or balanced salt medium, they will still be approximately

Table 3.6. Properties of iodixanol–sucrose solutions[a]

% Iodixanol (w/v)	η	ρ (g ml⁻¹)
10.00	1.3589	1.079
15.00	1.3659	1.103
20.00	1.3729	1.127
25.00	1.3799	1.151
30.00	1.3868	1.175
35.00	1.3938	1.199
40.00	1.4008	1.223
45.00	1.4078	1.248
50.00	1.4147	1.272

[a] 50% iodixanol working solution (see text) diluted with 0.25 M sucrose, 1 mM EDTA, 10 mM Tris–HCl, pH 7.4.
η, refractive index; ρ, density. The osmolality of the gradient solutions is in the range 295–310 mOsm.

Table 3.7. Properties of iodixanol–saline solutions[a]

% Iodixanol (w/v)	η	ρ (g ml^{-1})
10.00	1.3507	1.058
12.00	1.3538	1.069
14.00	1.3569	1.079
16.00	1.3601	1.090
18.00	1.3632	1.100
20.00	1.3663	1.111
22.00	1.3694	1.121
24.00	1.3726	1.132
26.00	1.3757	1.142
28.00	1.3788	1.153
30.00	1.3820	1.163
32.00	1.3851	1.174
34.00	1.3882	1.184
36.00	1.3914	1.195
38.00	1.3945	1.205
40.00	1.3976	1.215

[a] 40% iodixanol working solution (see text) diluted with 0.85% NaCl, 10 mM Tricine–NaOH, pH 7.4.
η, refractive index; ρ, density. The osmolality of the gradient solutions is in the range 285–300 mOsm.

isoosmotic, but the concentration of buffer and additives such as EDTA will not be constant.

Percoll®

Percoll® has little intrinsic osmotic activity; thus the normal practice is to produce a 90% (v/v) solution by mixing with an osmotic balancer of 10× the normal concentration to make it isoosmotic. These prepared solutions are called working stocks which can then be diluted with the normal concentration of osmotic balancer. For mammalian organelles, for example, the following solutions might be prepared.

■ Working stock of 90% (v/v) Percoll® is made by diluting 9 volumes of Percoll® with 1 volume of 2.5 M sucrose, 100 mM EDTA, 100 mM Tris–HCl, pH 7.4. The density of this solution is 1.149 g ml^{-1}. This is then further diluted with the HM (*Table 3.8*). The osmolality of the gradient solutions is 280–320 mOsm. Solutions for mammalian cells are prepared in a similar manner from a working stock of 9 volumes of Percoll® + 1 volume of 8.5% NaCl, 100 mM Tricine–NaOH, pH 7.4 which is further diluted with normal saline (*Table 3.9*).

For more details regarding gradient solutions for mammalian cells see Chapter 5 and Patel (2001).

Working solutions for non-mammalian organelles

Solutions for cells and organelles from non-mammalian sources are usually prepared at a higher osmolarities and often with other types of osmotic

Table 3.8. Properties of Percoll®–sucrose solutions[a]

% Percoll (w/v)	η	ρ (g ml^{-1})
10.00	1.3470	1.043
20.00	1.3490	1.056
30.00	1.3510	1.070
40.00	1.3530	1.083
50.00	1.3550	1.096
60.00	1.3570	1.109
70.00	1.3590	1.123
80.00	1.3610	1.135
90.00	1.3630	1.149

[a] 90% Percoll working solution (see text) diluted with 0.25 M sucrose, 1 mM EDTA, 10 mM Tris–HCl, pH 7.4.
η, refractive index; ρ, density. The osmolality of the gradient solutions is in the range 285–310 mOsm.

Table 3.9. Properties of Percoll®–NaCl solutions[a]

% Percoll (w/v)	η	ρ (g ml^{-1})
10.00	1.3368	1.018
20.00	1.3386	1.031
30.00	1.3405	1.044
40.00	1.3423	1.057
50.00	1.3442	1.071
60.00	1.3461	1.084
70.00	1.3479	1.096
80.00	1.3498	1.110
90.00	1.3516	1.123

[a] 90% Percoll working solution (see text) diluted with with 0.85% NaCl, 10 mM Tricine–NaOH, pH 7.4.
η, refractive index; ρ, density. The osmolality of the gradient solutions is in the range 285–310 mOsm.

balancers, consequently the working solutions and the osmotic balancers have to be prepared accordingly.

■ A working solution of 40% (w/v) iodixanol for yeast organelles might be prepared from 2 volumes of OptiPrep™ and 1 volume of 12.25% (w/v) sorbitol and then further diluted with 8.75% sorbitol. The density of these solutions is given in *Table 3.10* and their osmolality is approximately 550 mOsm.

4. Analysis of fractions

4.1 Compatibility of gradient media with analytical techniques

Ideally it should be possible to analyze a fraction from a gradient without prior removal of the medium. This not only eliminates possible losses of the particle but it is also a lot more convenient. Such a strategy is only possible if the concentration of the particle is sufficient to be analyzed effectively and if the medium does not interfere with the analytical technique, otherwise the fraction must be concentrated and the solute removed.

Table 3.10. Properties of iodixanol–sorbitol gradient solutions (approximately 550 mOsm)[a]

% Iodixanol (w/v)	η	ρ (g ml^{-1})
10.00	1.3596	1.078
15.00	1.3664	1.103
20.00	1.3736	1.127
25.00	1.3806	1.152
30.00	1.3878	1.176
35.00	1.3949	1.200
40.00	1.4020	1.225

[a] 40% iodixanol–sorbitol working solution diluted with 8.75% sorbitol (see text).
η, refractive index; ρ, density. The osmolality of the gradient solutions is in the range 545–560 mOsm.

Electrophoresis

None of the inorganic salts are compatible with any form of electrophoresis; consequently these media must be removed beforehand (Section 4.2). Percoll® also apparently interferes with the proper running of polyacrylamide gels. Low-molecular mass nonionic media (sucrose and all of the iodinated media, except diatrizaote and metrizoate) need not be removed, indeed they can replace the glycerol which is normally added to allow samples to be layered beneath running buffers.

Spectrophotometric assay

All of the true solutes, except the iodinated gradient media, are optically clear at visible and all useful ultraviolet (UV) wavelengths, i.e. protein and nucleic acids can be monitored at 260 and 280 nm, respectively. Because of the aromatic nucleus of metrizamide, Nycodenz® and iodixanol, these molecules absorb strongly in the UV region (*Figure 3.7*) and consequently fractions containing these media cannot be measured below approximately 360 nm. A major disadvantage of Percoll® is the requirement for its elimination prior to any spectrophotometric measurement (because of its light scattering properties). Moreover in this procedure, losses of organelles occurs (Section 4.2).

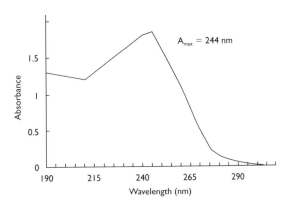

Figure 3.7

Absorbance profile of Nycodenz® (0.05 mg ml^{-1} in water).

Chemical assays

Any monosaccharide or polysaccharide containing medium (including metrizamide) is incompatible with nucleic acid assays which measure ribose or deoxyribose content (e.g. the orcinol and diphenylamine methods) spectrophotometrically. All iodinated density gradient media interfere with protein assays which measure amino groups or peptide bonds such as the Lowry and biuret assays (and sucrose interferes with the Lowry method, at high concentrations). However, if only small volumes of sample are used in the Lowry method so that the gradient solute is effectively diluted to less than 4% (w/v) by the assay solutions, then interference is minimal. Protein assays which employ Coomassie blue seem to be the least affected by any gradient medium.

Extraction with 2:1 chloroform/methanol, prior to lipid analysis, can be carried out on gradient fractions of any gradient medium directly. Gradient media will partition preferentially in the aqueous medium. Although high concentrations of inorganic salts may cause some of the more polar lipids to partition anomalously into the upper phase, these will be recovered when the upper phase is washed with water. Lipid analyses which are carried out on unextracted fractions such as the enzymic-chromogen-linked determination of cholesterol (Ahmed, 1993) may be inhibited by inorganic salts but not by nonionic media.

Enzyme assays

The majority of enzymes are assayed spectrophotometrically and the hence the same restrictions apply to the compatibility of gradient media as given above. In addition, some enzymes are inhibited by certain gradient media while some show a modest activation after exposure to the medium (*Table 3.11*). In all cases any inhibitory effects are reversible when the gradient medium is removed. The table compares sucrose, Nycodenz® and iodixanol only, as Percoll® has to be removed prior to assay (see above).

4.2   Removal of the gradient medium

If the biological particles are not sufficiently concentrated to be assayed accurately and/or if the gradient medium is incompatible with the analytic

Table 3.11. Effect of sucrose, Nycodenz® and iodixanol on some enzymes

Enzyme	Iodixanol	Nycodenz®	Sucrose
Succinate dehydrogenase	96; 103; 104	74; 87; 88	67; 90; 86
β-Galactosidase	101; 96; 102	93; 100; 100	95; 85; 77
Acid phosphatase	95; 101; 102	94; 102; 101	87; 93; 92
Alkaline phosphatase	143; 131; 135	152; 152; 152	115; 117; 112
Catalase	143; 140; 137	100; 91; 104	112; 111; 121
Mg^{2+}-ATPase	71; 74; 79	76; 77; 80	105; 84; 98
5'-Nucleotidase	109; 95; 99	96; 100; 98	91; 103; 97
NADPH-cyt c reductase	105; 112; 122	100; 108; 115	100; 113; 119
Leucine aminopeptidase	102; 88; 96	108; 100; 97	104; 93; 73

All figures are given as a percentage of the activity in the control medium (0.25 M sucrose, 1 mM EDTA, 20 mM Tricine–NaOH, pH 7.4). The three figures are the percentage activity after 0.5, 1.0 and 3.0 h incubation in 30% (w/v) medium.

cal procedure (Section 4.1), it may be necessary to pellet them and resuspend them in a smaller volume of a compatible medium. Carrying out this step also enables all the particles to be suspended in a medium of constant composition – undoubtedly beneficial to subsequent analysis but potentially a possible source of further loss of material and functional integrity.

Standard protocol

The most widely used procedure to harvest and concentrate particles from a gradient medium is to dilute the sample with two volumes of buffer (or suspension/ homogenization medium) in order to reduce the density and viscosity of the sample and then to centrifuge at an appropriate relative centrifugal field (RCF). If the density is not reduced then if the particle is banded isopycnically it will never sediment. Except for mammalian cells, the appropriate RCF should be slightly higher than the normal value used to pellet the particle in the pre-gradient procedure, since the medium will still be of a higher density and viscosity than the normal suspension/homogenization medium. For example, membrane vesicles which might normally be pelleted at 100 000 g for 40 min may require 150 000 g for the same (or longer) time. Ideally the pellet should not be so firmly packed that it requires excessive shearing forces to disaggregate it. A conical tube can be an advantage in that the pellet is more stable and clearly located.

Cells

Cells should be pelleted as gently as possible; more than 200–300 g should not be used. No gradient medium should provide any problems regarding effective and rapid removal. A number of cell types, however, may be deleteriously affected by any separation protocol; monocytes are particularly sensitive to handling and great care should be taken in resuspending pelleted material, otherwise they are readily activated.

Membrane vesicles and organelles

If the pellet is to be resuspended in a relatively small volume (e.g. 0.2 ml) losses of material in small homogenizers or syringes may be significant. In these instances it may be preferable to use vortex mixing. For the pelleting of organelles it is often convenient to use a microcentrifuge at 4°C in which samples can be rapidly pelleted (top speed for 15 min) in 1.0–1.5 ml microcentrifuge tubes; the pellets are then resuspended directly in a suitable enzyme assay medium and incubated after addition of substrate. For membrane vesicles a microultracentrifuge can provide a similar small volume facility, some Beckman and Sorvall fixed-angle rotors accommodating Eppendorf Safe-Lock™ polyallomer microcentrifuge tubes.

Percoll® poses a problem in that the RCFs used to pellet many biological particles are the same as those used to pellet the silica particles (50 000–100 000 g for 30–60 min). While cells pellet at much lower RCFs and do not present a problem, losses of organelles and membrane vesicles into the Percoll® pellet may be significant (Osmundsen, 1982). Sedimentation of the gradient medium is also sometimes encountered with iodixanol; this medium forms its own gradient in relatively high RCFs (>180 000 g for 3 h), thus pelleting of particles from iodixanol solutions should be carried out at no more than approximately 100 000 g for 1 h.

As an alternative to pelleting, dialysis or centrifugal ultrafiltration of gradient media (other than polysaccharides and Percoll®) may be used. Using the standard dialysis tubing, sucrose, inorganic salts and metrizamide dialyze readily, Nycodenz® slightly less readily and iodixanol only very slowly. Losses of material also tend to be incurred in dialysis bags.

Iodixanol and all the other low-molecular mass solutes can be effectively removed by ultrafiltration using Whatman VectaSpin Micro™ or VectaSpin 3™ centrifuge tube filters (or equivalent) and this is the preferred alternative to pelleting. These filters operate in a microcentrifuge and are particularly effective at concentrating samples containing macromolecules or macromolecular complexes; they have molecular weight cut-offs from 10 to 100 kDa.

Because of their high-molecular mass, polysaccharides cannot be removed from the sample material by dialysis or ultrafiltration; to remove the medium, biological particles must be recovered by diluting the gradient fractions and centrifugal pelleting.

Viruses

Pelleting and resuspension often leads to loss of infectivity and dialysis or ultrafiltration in microcentrifuge cones (see above) are regarded as superior methods (see above).

Nucleic acids, proteins and lipoproteins

Although, of the above methods, dialysis or ultrafiltration in microcentrifuge cones are the only valid ones, chemical precipitation is an alternative strategy.

References

Ahmed, H. (1993) Measurement of cholesterol in membranes. In: *Methods in Molecular Biology*, Vol. 19 (eds J.M. Graham and J.A. Higgins). Humana Press, Totowa, NJ, pp. 179–182.

Osmundsen, H. (1982) Factors which can influence β-oxidation by peroxisomes isolated from livers of clofibrate treated rats. Some properties of peroxisomal fractions isolated in a self-generated Percoll gradient by vertical rotor centrifugation. *Int. J. Biochem.* 14: 905–914.

Patel, D. (2001) Fractionation of cells by sedimentation methods. In: *Separating Cells*. BIOS Scientific Publishers Ltd, Oxford, pp. 48–86.

Pertoft, H., Rubin, K., Kjellen, L. and Klingerborn, L. (1977) The viability of cells grown or centrifuged in a new density gradient medium, Percoll. *Exp. Cell Res.* 110: 449–457.

Pertoft, H., Laurent, T.C., Laas, T. and Kagedal, L. (1978) Density gradients prepared from colloidal silica particles coated with polyvinylpyrrolidone (Percoll). *Anal. Biochem.* 88: 271–282.

Rickwood, D. (1984) The theory and practice of centrifugation. In: *Centrifugation – A Practical Approach* (ed. D. Rickwood). IRL Press at Oxford University Press, Oxford, pp. 1–43.

Rickwood, D. (1992) Centrifugal methods for characterizing macromolecules and their interactions. In: *Preparative Centrifugation – A Practical Approach* (ed. D. Rickwood). IRL Press at Oxford University Press, Oxford, pp. 143–186.

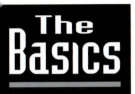

Chapter 4

Gradient techniques

1. Types of gradients and their uses

Unless the type of gradient for a particular preparative separation is well documented in the scientific literature, it is chosen largely empirically. A linear continuous gradient covering a broad range of densities is often the first choice in order to establish the banding density of the particle(s) of interest and that of any other contaminating particles. Subsequently it may be possible to devise a narrower range gradient to achieve a better resolution, or a discontinuous gradient to achieve a simpler separation. Banding of a particle at an interface is often considered to be an advantage for preparative purposes inasmuch as any band will be sharply defined and more easily recovered on a routine basis, but its purity may be sacrificed.

Analytical gradients which are used, for example, to study the sedimentation properties of proteins, are always continuous linear gradients. Linear gradients are also widely used to analyze processes such as endocytosis or secretion in which macromolecules are processed by the cell during their translocation through a number of membrane compartments, which can be distinguished from one another only by relatively small differences in density. These minor differences virtually preclude any attempt to purify some compartments in a pure form (e.g. the various domains of the Golgi or ER-*cis* Golgi transport vesicles) but such a gradient does permit the study of the translocation process during which a macromolecule or macromolecular complex is sequentially assembled or modified within each of these compartments. Some protocols to analyze these processes employ multistep discontinuous rather than continuous gradients for fine fractionation. This is technically difficult on a frequent routine basis. The density discontinuities in such gradients become smoothed out with time due to the diffusion of the gradient solute; indeed diffusion of such gradients is often used as a method of preparing continuous gradients (Section 3.1). Discontinuous gradients containing a large number of small-volume steps will approach linearity much more rapidly than those containing a small number of large-volume steps. During relatively short centrifugations, however (e.g. 3 h at 4°C), the gradients will retain some degree of discontinuity, and this can sharpen the banding of some compartments.

Gradients of some media (sucrose, potassium bromide, Ficoll, dextran) have to be made in a pre-formed manner, that is the operator must prepare them in the centrifuge tube prior to centrifugation. Pre-formed gradients can be made before the sample is applied either to the top of the gradient in a low-density medium or at the bottom of the gradient in a high-density medium. They can also be made such that the sample is incorporated into one or more of the density solutions that are used. Other gradient media

(Nycodenz®, iodixanol, CsCl, Percoll®) also offer the ability to be created by the centrifugal field (self-generated), that is they are formed in the spinning rotor from a medium of uniform density which contains the sample. Occasionally the gradient may be self-generated before the sample is applied (see Chapter 8). Self-generated gradients offer simplicity of preparation and very high reproducibility, as their formation and the gradient density profile that is produced depends solely on the centrifugation time, RCF, temperature and starting concentration of the gradient solute.

2.   Pre-formed discontinuous gradients

2.1   Overlayering technique

The most widely used method for producing discontinuous gradients is to start with the densest solution and layer successively lower densities on top from a pipette (*Figure 4.1*). The higher the viscosity of the medium, the easier it is to achieve a relatively slow and smooth flow of liquid from the pipette, while very low-density solutions, especially those of inorganic salts, are more difficult. A syringe with a wide-bore metal filling cannula (i.d. 1–2 mm) can be used as an alternative to a pipette. If the gradient solution is pre-measured, it may be applied from a Pasteur pipette, but practice is required in achieving a slow smooth flow of liquid when the bulb is gently depressed.

Practical tips when overlayering from a pipette

1. When layering one solution on top of another from a pipette, use a rubber two- or three-valve pipette filler to fill and dispense the gradient solutions.
2. Check that the release valve, when pressed gently, allows the delivery of a slow and steady flow of liquid.
3. Do not use a pipette filler which uses positive pressure to deliver the liquid as a slow even flow is often difficult to attain.
4. Always take up more of the gradient medium than is required for the step as it is easier and more accurate to empty the pipette to a graduation mark than to try to empty it completely.

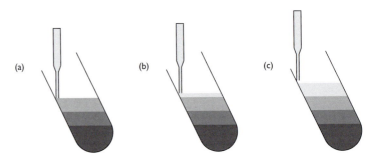

Figure 4.1

Construction of a discontinuous gradient by overlayering. (a) Place tip of pipette containing lower-density solution at junction of meniscus and wall of tilted tube. (b) Allow liquid to flow slowly and smoothly on to denser layer, keeping the pipette tip at the rising meniscus. (c) Withdraw the pipette against the wall of the tube.

5. Place the tip of the pipette at the meniscus of the denser layer against the wall of the tube and keep it at the rising meniscus of the new layer.

Practical tips when overlayering from a syringe

1. Make sure that the barrel can move easily and smoothly when a small pressure is applied.
2. Always take up more of the gradient medium than is required for the step as it is more accurate to empty the syringe to a graduation mark than to try to empty it completely.
3. Place the tip of the cannula at the wall of the centrifuge tube a couple of centimetres above the meniscus of the denser layer and gently press the plunger. This allows the liquid to spread over the tube surface and minimizes any mixing due to a sudden movement of the plunger. It may be useful to tilt the tube slightly.
4. Once a steady flow is established keep the tip of the cannula at the meniscus of the liquid and against the wall of the tube.

Practical tips when overlayering from a Pasteur pipette

1. With the tube slightly tilted, place the tip of the pipette a couple of centimetres above the meniscus of the denser solution against the wall of the tube and gently press the bulb to deliver a slow and steady stream of liquid.

2.2 Underlayering technique

Although the overlayering technique is probably the most widely used, the method in which successively denser solutions are underlayered under lighter ones is certainly the easier and the recommended one. The only important requirement is that no air bubbles are introduced which may disturb the lower density layers above; for this reason a syringe with a metal filling cannula is the best tool for this procedure. Generally, less disturbance to the existing steps is produced as the outflowing liquid spreads upwards through the hemispherical section of the bottom of the tube. Again the more viscous solutions are generally more easy to handle.

Practical tips

1. To layer 4 ml of liquid, take up 5 ml into the syringe and expel to the 4.5 ml mark to ensure that the cannula is full of liquid. Then dry the outside of the cannula.
2. Place the tip of the cannula at the bottom of the tube (slide it slowly down the wall of the tube) and depress the plunger to the 0.5 ml mark (*Figure 4.2*).
3. After a few seconds (to allow all of the liquid to be delivered into the tube) slowly withdraw the cannula, again against the wall of the tube (*Figure 4.2*).

In any of these pre-formed discontinuous gradients, the sample can subsequently either be layered on top in a low-density solution or at the bottom in a high-density solution once the gradient has been formed or it may be incorporated into any or all of the density steps.

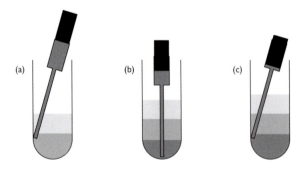

Figure 4.2

Construction of a discontinuous gradient by underlayering. To layer 5 ml of next dense solution, draw 6 ml into syringe and expel liquid to 5.5 ml mark. (a) Introduce tip of cannula to bottom of tube down wall of tube. (b) Move tip of cannula to center and gently expel the liquid to the 0.5 ml mark. (c) Withdraw the cannula against the wall of the tube. This procedure ensures no air bubbles are introduced with the dense liquid.

3.   Pre-formed continuous gradients

Continuous gradients may be made using a gradient maker specifically designed for this purpose or by allowing discontinuous gradients to diffuse.

3.1   By diffusion of discontinuous gradients

Once a discontinuous gradient is formed, the sharp boundaries between the layers which are observed as a sudden change in refractive index, start to disappear as the solute molecules diffuse down the concentration gradient from each denser layer to each lighter layer. Thus the density discontinuities between each layer will slowly even out and the gradient will eventually become linear (*Figure 4.3*) and given sufficient time the density will become completely uniform.

For a particular medium, the rate of diffusion across an interface is dependent on temperature and the cross-sectional area of the interface. In addition the rate at which the gradient becomes linear will also be a function of the distance between the interfaces. Thus a linear gradient will form

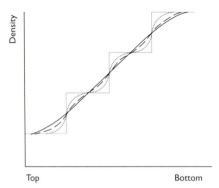

Figure 4.3

Formation of a continuous density gradient by diffusion of a discontinuous gradient. Profile of discontinuous gradient (——), diffusion smooths out discontinuities (dashed and dotted lines) to form continuous gradient (——).

more rapidly at room temperature than at 4°C and if the distance between interfaces is reduced and their cross-sectional area increased. This can be achieved by carefully rotating the sealed tube from a vertical to a horizontal position. For example, under these conditions (and at room temperature) a discontinuous gradient of say 10, 15, 20 and 25% (w/v) iodixanol (for example, 4 ml each in a 17-ml tube) will become linear in about 40 min. The tube is then rotated carefully back to its vertical position. These two reorientations, if carried out smoothly, produce surprisingly little mixing.

■   Whether the tube is filled to the top or includes a column of air above the liquid seems to make very little difference to continuous gradient formation.

Although formation of a linear gradient will occur more rapidly with the tube in a horizontal position, diffusion is often carried out in a vertical tube. A convenient approach is to prepare the discontinuous gradients the day before the experiment at room temperature and then to leave in the refrigerator overnight. As a general rule this is satisfactory for most 14–38 ml tubes for swinging-bucket rotors; 5 ml tubes will require 5–8 h depending on layer volume and viscosity.

Whichever strategy is adopted, the precise timing will depend on the dimensions of the tube, the number of layers and the concentrations of solute. A series of trial experiments should be carried out in which the time is varied and the density profile of the formed gradient checked by fractionation and refractive index measurement.

■   Remember that diffusion will continue during the subsequent centrifugation run.

Because the continuous gradient is formed by a physical process, then as long as the temperature and time are well controlled, the shape of the gradient is highly reproducible.

The sample may be applied to the gradient after diffusion or it may be incorporated into one or more of the layers before diffusion. Only when diffusion is carried out in a horizontal tube at room temperature is the latter a useful practice; thus this is normally restricted to the fractionation of some cell types.

3.2. By freeze–thawing

There are two major advantages of this technique: (i) its simplicity and (ii) centrifuge tubes, filled with the appropriate solution, can be stored frozen until required. However, it is not recommended for the production of isoosmotic gradients (Chapter 3), using, for example, NaCl as an osmotic balancer, because the distribution of ions within the gradient after thawing cannot be easily predicted. However, if the aim is to produce a gradient merely containing additives such as an organic buffer and EDTA, whose concentrations through the gradient are not particularly important, then this procedure is worth considering. Although the density-gradient profile is very dependent on tube volume and the rates of freezing and thawing, if these procedures are carried out in a controlled and reproducible manner, then the shape of the gradient that is formed will also be highly reproducible. The actual shape of the density profile also depends to some extent on the type and concentration of the gradient solute. Gradient shape can also be influenced by the number of freeze–thaw cycles and as the number increases so the gradients become less dense at the top, more dense at the bottom and less shallow in the middle of the tube.

The profiles of iodixanol gradients shown in *Figure 4.4* were obtained in 5 ml tubes; freezing to $-20°C$ took approximately 30 min and thawing at room temperature occurred in 30–60 min. Further freezing was commenced within 30 min of complete thawing.

3.3 Using a two-chamber gradient maker

The traditional method of constructing a continuous gradient is to use a standard two-chamber gradient maker (*Figure 4.5*). It consists of two identical chambers connected close to their bases by a tapped channel. One of the chambers (the mixing chamber) has an outlet directly opposite the inlet from the tapped channel. The device is set up with the mixing chamber resting on a magnetic stirrer and the outlet tube leading, via a peristaltic pump, to the bottom of the centrifuge tube.

Practical tips

1. Place the chosen high-density solution in the non-mixing chamber and open the tap momentarily to fill the connecting tube.
2. Place an equal volume of the low density solution in the mixing chamber.
3. Place two identical stirring bars in the two chambers to ensure that the height of the two solutions is the same.
4. Always start the procedure in this order: switch the pump on, start the magnetic stirrer and open the connecting tap.
5. As the levels in the two chambers fall synchronously, reduce the speed of the stirrer to avoid generating air bubbles which may enter the gradient and disturb it.
6. The larger the density difference between the two gradient solutions the more vigorous must be the stirring to ensure good mixing.

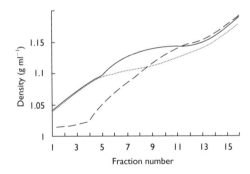

Figure 4.4

Formation of a continuous density gradient by freeze–thawing. In 5-ml tubes, a solution of 20% iodixanol frozen to $-20°C$ for 30 min and then allowed to thaw at room temperature. One freeze–thaw cycle (·······); two cycles (——); three cycles (– –). C.A. Bornecque, CNRS, 91198 Gif sur Yvette, France, personal communication.

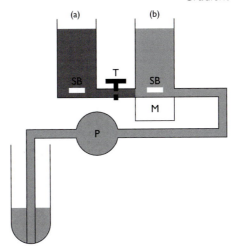

Figure 4.5

A two-chamber continuous gradient maker. With low-density solution in the mixing chamber (b) and dense solution (a), liquid of linearly increasing density is delivered to the bottom of the centrifuge tube. T, tap; SB, stirring bar; P, peristaltic pump; M, magnetic stirrer.

7. If the stirring bar is too close to the inlet from the connecting tube, it is possible in the initial stages for the low-density medium to back-flow into the high-density medium.

8. The correct pumping speed depends on the volume of the gradient and the quality of the pump (ideally the outflow from the pump should not pulsate), but for a standard gradient (12–15 ml total volume) a flow rate of 2–3 ml min^{-1} is satisfactory.

The gradient can alternatively be produced high-density end first, in which case the location of the two solutions needs to be reversed and the delivery tube to the centrifuge tube must be placed against the wall of the tube near to its top, so the gradient flows down the tube smoothly. This can pose some problems of mixing in the centrifuge tube if the flow down the tube wall is in the form of large drops rather than a continuous stream; on the other hand, the tendency of the low-density medium to float to the surface of the high-density medium in the mixing chamber may aid good mixing (see Section 6.6).

It is possible to produce up to three gradients at a time; some gradient mixers have a three-outlet manifold. However, such a device requires three tubes to pass through the peristaltic pump. It is, however, the only reliable configuration of the delivery tube: simply splitting a single effluent from the pump into three streams does not guarantee precisely equal delivery to the three tubes.

3.4 The Gradient Master®

An alternative device for the generation of continuous density gradients – the Gradient Master® – produces the gradient by controlled mixing of the low- and high-density solutions layered in the centrifuge tube. The tubes are rotated at a pre-set angle – usually 80° – to increase the cross-sectional area of the interface – and speed (usually 20 r.p.m.) for about 2 min (*Figure 4.6*).

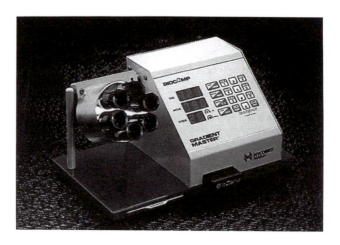

Figure 4.6

Gradient Master® continuous gradient maker. The photograph shows six 14 ml tubes being rotated at 80° (see text for details). From Biocomp Instruments Inc, Fredricton, NB, Canada.

The density profile of the gradient generally becomes more shallow with time. The simplicity of the technique and the highly reproducible nature of the gradients make this a very attractive method particularly as up to six gradients (17 ml tubes) can be formed at once. Some examples of iodixanol gradients are given in *Figure 4.7*.

A very important advantage of this technique over the use of a two-chamber gradient mixer is that if it is necessary to make the sample part of the gradient, any potentially hazardous biological sample is contained within the centrifuge tube and does not contaminate any gradient-forming device and ancillary tubing.

3.5   Temperature control

If pre-formed gradients are produced which already incorporate the sample, then they must be formed at the temperature used for the centrifugation. Gradients made at room temperature must be allowed to reach the temper-

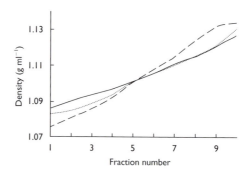

Figure 4.7

Density profiles of gradients produced by Gradient Master®. Profiles produced from 7 ml each of 10 and 40% (w/v) iodixanol, rotated at 20 r.p.m., at 80° for (− −) 2 min, (······) 2.5 min and (——) 3 min.

ature at which they are to be centrifuged before applying the sample. Many cell types (particularly blood cells) are often centrifuged at room temperature, but cells from enzymically disaggregated tissues and most other biological particles tend to be fractionated at 4°C, although plasma lipoproteins are commonly centrifuged at 16°C. Rotors and rotor chambers should also be pre-cooled to the operational temperature. The larger the gradient volume the longer it will take to reach temperature equilibrium and particularly during short runs (less than 3 h) at 4°C, if the gradients and hardware are not pre-cooled, the gradients may never reach the desired temperature.

4. Nonlinear gradients

It is not always desirable to use a linear gradient and either convex, concave, S-shaped or more complex gradient-density profiles (*Figure 4.8*) may be required to effect a particular resolution of particles. Convex gradients are sometimes particularly useful for the resolution of a sample containing a high concentration of particles of a wide range of densities. The steep density profile at the top of the gradient provides stable conditions for high capacity and the shallower high-density region provides high resolution.

A shallow gradient may be effective in resolving particles of similar density but more often it simply results in band broadening rather than any improvement in resolving power. Band broadening can, however, be useful if the particle under investigation displays some evidence of functional or compositional heterogeneity with density. Individual populations of most biological particles, particularly cells, organelles, membrane vesicles, viruses and major classes of plasma lipoproteins have a heterogeneous nature and display ranges of densities rather than a single defined density. However, hydrostatic or hydrodynamic instability problems may also be responsible for broad bands (see Chapter 1).

S-shaped profiles which contain a very shallow central section may be of particular use for resolving two different particles of rather similar density. However, if such an approach is designed to establish that there are two subpopulations of the same particle, the presence of two peaks of particle

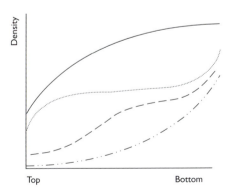

Figure 4.8

Nonlinear density gradient profiles. Convex gradient (——), concave gradient (— ··), S-shaped gradient (········), complex gradient (— —).

activity on either side of a shallow central region of an S-shaped gradient may not be a true indication of the existence of two distinct subpopulations. The biphasic distribution may simply be caused by gradient shape if the band is distributed across a shallow region between two steep gradients. *Figure 4.9* shows the distribution of a lysosome marker in a Percoll® gradient plotted as marker concentration versus volume of gradient, suggesting two bands of organelles. If the data is replotted as frequency (amount of marker divided by the density interval covered by each fraction) against density then a single peak is obtained (*Figure 4.9*). The two-band artifact is created by heterogeneity of particle density combined with the gradient shape (Draye *et al.*, 1987).

More complex shapes combining a series of steep and shallow gradient regions may provide very specific solutions to some separation problems but these need to be worked out empirically for each situation.

4.1   Nonlinear gradients by diffusion

The diffusion of discontinuous gradients method is a very convenient way of producing a gradient that is not linear with volume. By gradually increasing or decreasing the volume of each step, the gradient will assume a curved form (concave or convex) and if the volume of a single intermediate layer is increased then a shallow median section will be introduced into the continuous gradient. As with linear gradients, it is important to test the density profile that is formed from such discontinuous gradients, but once satisfactory conditions are established, the profile will be highly reproducible.

4.2   Nonlinear gradients using a two-chamber gradient maker

Convex and concave gradients cannot be produced with the standard two-chamber gradient mixer. If, however, the non-mixing chamber is made twice the diameter of the mixing chamber, then with low-density solution in the

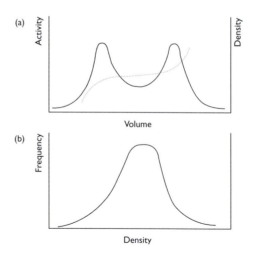

Figure 4.9

Artifactual banding of particles caused by gradient-density shape. (a) In an S-shaped gradient (dotted line) the distribution of an activity (% of total) vs. tube volume produces a biphasic distribution. (b) When replotted as a frequency (activity per density interval) a Gaussian distribution is obtained.

mixing chamber a convex gradient is produced and if the locations of the low-density and high-density solutions are reversed, then a concave gradient is produced. Another simple means of producing a convex gradient is to use a constant mixing volume gradient mixer of the type shown in *Figure 4.10*. In this closed system, the volume of gradient solution removed from the mixing chamber by the pump is replaced by an equal volume of dense solution delivered into the mixing chamber from the reservoir.

The actual shape of the density profile produced by the two devices is slightly different – that produced by the adapted two-chamber gradient maker tends to be less steep (and closer to a linear form) in the lower-density region of a convex gradient than that produced by a constant mixing volume gradient maker. *Figure 4.11* compares the calculated density-gradient profiles of a 30-ml 10–20% (w/v) gradient of a solute prepared from 20 ml of 20% and 10 ml of 10% solute in an adapted two-chamber gradient maker, and 30 ml of 20% solute added to 10 ml of 10% solute in a constant mixing volume gradient maker. When calculating the conditions necessary to produce a convex (or concave) gradient always remember that in the constant mixing volume gradient maker, 10 ml of the low-density (or high-density) solution remain in the mixing chamber at the end of the gradient formation, while in the case of the adapted two-chamber gradient maker, all of the two solutions are used up.

Gradients with more complex density profiles cannot be easily produced by any of the simple gradient makers. Formation from a discontinuous gradient would be relatively simple but many trial runs would be needed to achieve the desired gradient shape; however, once a system had been found, it would be highly reproducible. A programmable gradient maker is the only real alternative, but they are expensive and not always suited to the large volumes of sometimes viscous media.

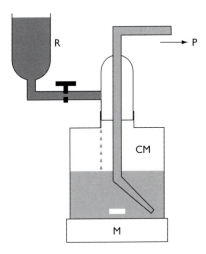

Figure 4.10

Constant-volume convex gradient maker. R, Reservoir containing dense solution; CM, closed constant-volume mixing chamber containing low-density solution; M, magnetic stirrer; P, peristaltic pump.

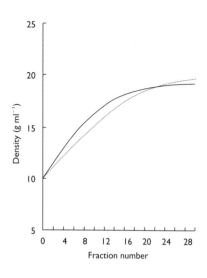

Figure 4.11

Density profiles of convex gradients. Produced by modified two-chamber maker (·······), and constant-volume mixer (——).

See Chapter 2 for information regarding the types of rotors used for pre-formed density gradients.

5.   Self-generating gradients

5.1   A brief summary of the theory

Solutions of heavy metal salts (e.g. CsCl) and the iodinated density-gradient media (particularly iodixanol) can form a gradient from a solution of uniform density under the influence of the centrifugal field. Once the solute begins to sediment through the solvent, a concentration gradient is formed which is opposed by back-diffusion of the solute. With a sufficiently high relative centrifugal field (RCF), at equilibrium, the sedimentation of the solute is exactly balanced by the diffusion and the gradient is stable. It is possible to calculate the time for a self-generating gradient to reach equilibrium and it is described by Equation 4.1.

$$t = k(r_b - r_t)^2 \tag{4.1}$$

where t is the time in hours; r_b and r_t is the distance from the center of rotation to the bottom and top of the gradient respectively and k is a constant which depends on the diffusion coefficient and viscosity of the solute and on temperature (Dobrota and Hinton, 1992). The slope of the gradient is given by Equation 4.2;

$$\rho_r = \rho_i - \frac{1.1 \times 10^{-2} \times Q^2}{2\beta^0}(r^2_c - r^2) \tag{4.2}$$

where ρ_r is the density at a point r cm from the axis of rotation, ρ_i is the starting density of the homogeneous solution, r_c is the distance in centimeters from the axis of rotation where the density of the gradient = ρ_i, Q is the rotor speed in r.p.m. and β^0 is a constant depending on the properties of the solute. There are a number of texts which give values for these constants. In many cases, however, the centrifugation conditions required to generate a particular gradient-density profile can be more simply deduced from published data. For more information on the theoretical aspects of self-generated gradient formation, see Hames (1984), Dobrota and Hinton (1992) and Rickwood (1992).

5.2   Factors influencing the density profile of gradients

While the density range of the gradient that is formed is a function of the starting concentration of the solute the density profile of the gradient for any particular solute depends on the following operational parameters:

- sedimentation path-length of the rotor;
- time of centrifugation;
- speed of centrifugation;
- temperature.

Changing these factors affects the shape of the gradient in much the same manner, irrespective of the gradient medium, although the precise conditions required to form a particular density profile will clearly vary with the solute. For heavy metal salts and iodinated density-gradient media, the RCFs that are required are above 100 000 g, and for efficient gradient formation in relatively short times (3–6 h) RCFs of above 300 000 g are more commonly used.

The effects of changing the sedimentation path length of the rotor, centrifugation time and RCF can be predicted by Equations 4.1 and 4.2. It is, however, beyond the scope of this book to present a detailed analysis of the behavior of solute molecules in a centrifugal field, and comment will be confined principally to a few illustrative examples of how each of the above parameters affects the density profile of iodixanol gradients.

Figures 4.12–4.15 compare the gradient profiles of iodixanol gradients formed in vertical, near-vertical and fixed-angle rotors under a variety of centrifugation conditions and a comparison of these gradient profiles will reveal the following.

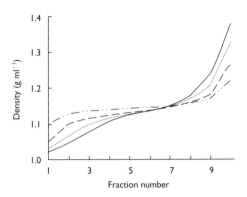

Figure 4.12

Self-generated gradients of iodixanol (in 0.85% saline) in the Sorvall S150-AT fixed-angle rotor (2 ml): effect of time of centrifugation. Centrifugation at 150 000 r.p.m. (16°C) for 15 min (— ··), 30 min (– –), 45 min (·······) and 60 min (—).

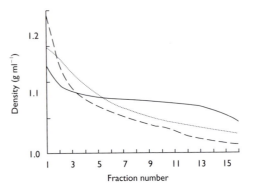

Figure 4.13

Self-generated gradients of iodixanol (in 0.85% saline) in the Beckman TLN100 near-vertical rotor (3.1 ml): effect of time. Centrifugation at 353 000 g and 16°C for 1 h (——); 2 h (······); 3 h (– –).

1. At the shortest time of centrifugation, the density profile of the gradient is more or less S-shaped (*Figure 4.12*). In the limiting situation, this central section is more or less flat and extends almost throughout the gradient. As the time increases, so this central section becomes steeper; the density towards the top decreases and consequently the profile becomes almost linear over much of the gradient (*Figure 4.12*). The profiles in *Figure 4.12* were obtained with one of the highest performance small-volume rotors that is currently available – a Sorvall fixed-angle rotor (S150–AT) with a sedimentation path-length of only 15 mm which can generate approx 1 000 000 g_{max} when run at 150 000 r.p.m.

2. The Beckman TLN100 near-vertical rotor has a very similar path-length (17 mm) but has a lower maximum RCF. An identical effect of time is observed but since the rotor is run at a lower RCF the actual times required are longer (*Figure 4.13*). The density at the very bottom of the gradient increases markedly with time and, depending on the rotor

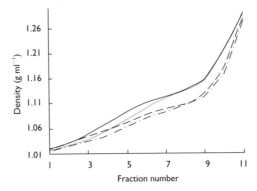

Figure 4.14

Self-generated gradients of iodixanol (in 0.25 M sucrose) in the Beckman VTi65.1 vertical rotor (11.2 ml): effect of time and iodixanol concentration. Centrifugation at 353 000 g (4°C): 15% iodixanol (– –) 4 h, (— ·) 5 h; 20% iodixanol (——) 4 h, (······) 5 h.

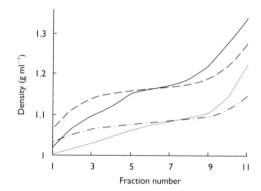

Figure 4.15

Self-generated gradients of iodixanol (in 0.85% NaCl) in the Beckman VTi65.1 vertical rotor (11.2 ml): effect of RCF and iodixanol concentration. Centrifugation at 353 000 g (16°C): 15% iodixanol (—·) 170 000 g, (·······) 353 000 g; 30% iodixanol (– –) 170 000 g, (——) 353 000 g.

type and the RCF, the gradient may eventually become almost exponential being very shallow at the top.

3. At a particular RCF the gradient will, given sufficient time, reach equilibrium at which the rate of sedimentation of the solute is exactly balanced by its rate of back-diffusion and the density profile will stabilize. In the Beckman VTi65.1 vertical rotor this time is 4–5 h at maximum speed (*Figure 4.14*).

4. Increasing the RCF while maintaining a set centrifugation time achieves a similar effect to increasing the time at a set RCF, that is, the gradient density profile changes from S-shaped to become more or less linear (*Figure 4.15*) over most of its length.

5. The effect of increased path length is shown in *Figure 4.16*, which shows the density profiles from a fixed-angle rotor (Beckman 80Ti) with a

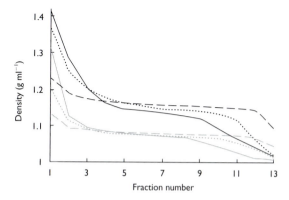

Figure 4.16

Self-generated gradients of iodixanol (in 0.85% NaCl) in the Beckman 80Ti fixed-angle rotor (13.5 ml): effect of time and iodixanol concentration. Centrifugation at 340 000 g (16°C): 15% iodixanol (– –) 1.5 h, (·······) 5 h, (——) 7h; 30% iodixanol (– –) 1.5 h, (·······) 5 h, (——) 7 h.

sedimentation path-length of nearly 40 mm. Even after 5 h at 340 000 g the gradient profile is clearly S-shaped, only approaching linearity in the top half of the gradient after 7 h.

6. Gradients tend to form rather more rapidly at higher temperatures but the effect is fairly marginal and more apparent at shorter times of 1 h than at longer times of centrifugation.

Thus although vertical and near-vertical rotors may be the rotors of choice for self-generated gradients, fixed-angle rotors, particularly those with a low angle ($20-24°$) and small tube volume (<10 ml), may be satisfactory. Larger-volume fixed-angle rotors may require at least 15 h before a useful gradient is formed. On the other hand, the modern small-volume high-performance fixed-angle rotors can form useful gradients in less than 1 h. Rotors with a sedimentation path-length of less than approximately 23 mm are ideal for self-generated gradients; those with path lengths above 35 mm are much less suitable.

Swinging-bucket rotors, which tend to have the longest sedimentation path-lengths, are almost never used as such for self-generated gradients; their density profiles never change from S-shaped. However, some of the Beckman fixed-angle and all of the swinging-bucket rotors can be modified with g-Max adaptors (Chapter 2) to accommodate smaller-volume tubes with reduced sedimentation path-lengths. In this manner some of these rotors may be converted to a format which is suitable for self-generated gradient.

Percoll®

Percoll® also forms its own gradients under the influence of the centrifugal field but since it is a colloidal suspension of silica particles, this occurs at much lower RCFs than with true solutes such as CsCl or iodixanol. Moreover, establishment of a gradient with Percoll® occurs in a slightly different manner. Due to the presence of a range of silica particle size, the larger ones sediment ahead of the smaller ones. Thus, from an initially uniform dispersion of particles a gradient will form. RCFs in the range 20 000–100 000 g for 20–40 min are commonly used (*Figure 4.17*). Although the manner in which a Percoll® gradient is formed by the centrifugal field is rather different from that of the other media, the effects of the various centrifugation parameters on gradient shape are broadly similar. The series of profiles in *Figure 4.17* demonstrates one of the inherent problems of Percoll® which is that even at relatively low RCFs the silica particles may sediment before the membranes have been able to reach their banding density. The rapid change in density profile may also be inconvenient.

■ Vertical rotors are never used with self-generated Percoll® gradients since some of the colloidal particles often sediment onto the wall of the tube.

6. Harvesting gradients

The mode of harvesting depends very much on the type of tube used for the gradient, the distribution of particles in the gradient and the aim of the fractionation. There are five main modes of gradient harvesting. *Table 4.1* summarizes the unloading modes which are compatible with different types of tube.

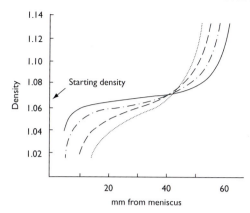

Figure 4.17

Self-generated gradients of Percoll (in 0.85% NaCl) in a 14 ml fixed-angle rotor at 20 000 g: effect of time. Starting density = 1.07 g ml^{-1}; (——) 15 min; (— ·) 30 min, (— —) 60 min, (·······) 90 min.

6.1   Harvesting single or multiple bands

If the banded material is clearly observable and well resolved then the tip of a cannula (attached to a syringe) or Pasteur pipette (preferably fashioned into an L-shape) can be placed in the band and the material withdrawn. The band can only be effectively removed in a small volume if the tip of the cannula or pipette can be moved around horizontally in the band, thus narrow-necked or sealed tubes are more difficult to handle.

This method can be used to harvest the entire gradient, if the tip of the pipette or cannula is placed at the meniscus. It is, however, tedious, prone to error and difficult to obtain equal volume fractions (if that is a requirement), but for a crude fractionation into four or five regions it is quite satisfactory.

6.2   Aspiration using a peristaltic pump

As a general rule, the harvesting system should be devised so that the effluent from the tube should not have to pass through a pump, but as long as the dead volume of the tubing is small compared to the volume of the gradient, it is permissible to insert a narrow tube to the bottom of the centrifuge tube and to aspirate the contents (dense end first). Theoretically, mixing will occur in the vertical section of the collection tubing as the decreasingly dense medium enters the bottom of the tube. In practice, however, this seems not to be a serious problem.

6.3   By tube puncture

If the tube is thin-walled, it is possible to puncture the bottom of the tube with a hollow needle; this is particularly easy with the softer polyallomer tubes, but impractical with thick walled tubes and it is not a useful method if there is a large pellet which may obstruct the hollow needle. It is best carried out by securing the tube vertically in some form of clamping device and to advance the needle through a rubber seal into the bottom of the tube by a screw or lever mechanism (*Figure 4.18*). The Beckman Fraction Recovery

Table 4.1. Suitability of ultracentrifuge tube type for different types of unloading

Tube type	Recommended method[a]	Comments and problems
Open-topped, thin-walled	Tube puncture Upward displacement Tube slicing Aspiration (dense end first) Automatic from meniscus	
Open-topped, thick-walled	Upward displacement Aspiration (dense end first) Automatic from meniscus	Collection head must be sealed onto top of tube with a rubber gasket.
Screw-capped, thick-walled	Upward displacement Aspiration (dense end first) Automatic from meniscus	Collection head must be sealed onto top of tube with a rubber gasket. Material can get trapped at the shoulders of the tube
Sealed (heat or crimp)	Tube puncture Tube slicing *Aspiration (dense end first)* *Automatic from meniscus*	 The tube must be sliced at the neck, this must be performed with great care. Same problems as above.
Sealed (Optiseal™, Re-seal™ or Easy-seal™)	Tube puncture Upward displacement Tube slicing Aspiration (dense end first) Aspiration from meniscus	 The dense unloading medium is best introduced by tube puncture. The effluent from the top of the tube is collected by sealing a narrow delivery tube into the neck of the centrifuge tube. Check that the collection head can enter the tube unimpeded by the neck.

[a] Methods which pose some degree of risk to the operator and to the stability of the gradient are *italicized*.

System incorporates such a device. Tops of heat-sealed or crimp-sealed tubes must also be punctured with a syringe needle to allow air to displace the descending liquid. In the most recent types of sealed tube (Beckman Optiseal™, Sorvall Easy-Seal™ and Re-Seal™, the central plastic plug may simply be removed.

The tube puncture system is simple and the dead space of the collecting tube (the bore of the needle) is almost negligible. Also the hemispherical section of the bottom of the tube directs banded material into the collecting needle, making gradient collection almost ideal. However, if the densest part of the gradient is very viscous, the initial collection rate by gravity may be very slow. This process can be speeded up by inserting a peristaltic pump

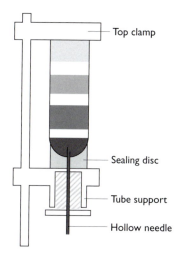

Figure 4.18

Gradient unloading by tube puncture. Tube held vertically between top clamp and sealing disc mounted on tube support. Modern versions use a pivoted lever to advance the hollow needle rather than the screw-thread shown.

into the collection line and small modern pumps and narrow bore tubing can avoid unacceptable increases in the dead space of the collection tubing and, with a suitable fraction collector, the process can improve the ease and reliability of fraction collection.

■   If a fraction collector is used in a 'number of drops' mode the volume of the fractions will change as the drop size is affected by the viscosity and surface tension of the liquid.

It is possible to collect a specific band within the gradient by puncturing a sealed tube with a needle attached to a syringe just below the band and with the inlet to the needle uppermost, aspirating the band into the syringe (*Figure 4.19*). As with bottom puncture, air must be allowed to displace the falling column of liquid in the tube.

6.4   By upward displacement

If a dense liquid can be introduced to the bottom of the tube then the gradient can be displaced upwards and collected from open topped thin-walled tubes for swinging-bucket rotors. A cylindrical block of clear acrylic, which fits into the top of the tube, contains a central channel which connects with a hollow cone (*Figure 4.20*). A side arm in the block connects with the central channel. The dense unloading solution is introduced to the bottom of the centrifuge tube from a long metal cannula. The gradient is displaced upwards by the incoming dense medium into the cone and an 'O'-ring around the cannula diverts the flow into the side arm and collection tubes (*Figures 4.20* and *4.21*). If the collector is alternatively sealed on to the top of the tube under pressure via a gasket (e.g Beckman Fraction Recovery System), this method can also be used on thick-walled tubes.

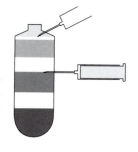

Figure 4.19

Removal of a band of material from a sealed tube using a syringe. The empty top syringe allows ingress of air to displace the gradient.

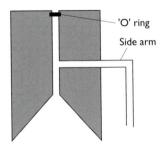

Figure 4.20

Home-made gradient unloader (upward displacement). See Figure 4.21.

Practical tips

1. Set up a buret with tubing connected via a peristaltic pump to the top of the metal cannula of the unloading device (*Figure 4.21*).
2. Place a dense unloading medium in a buret. Maxidens™ a non-water miscible, low-viscosity, high-density solution ($\rho = 1.9$ g ml^{-1}) is the best medium.
3. Using the pump, fill the tubing and cannula with the dense medium and adjust its level in the buret to a suitable graduation mark.
4. Wipe off any liquid at the tip of the cannula and insert it smoothly through the central channel to the bottom of the tube.
5. Restart the pump and collect the fractions from the side arm. The rate of gradient unloading should be approximately 2 ml min^{-1}.

This method facilitates the collection of fractions of known volume.

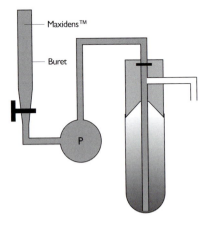

Figure 4.21

Gradient unloading by upward displacement. Unloader (see Figure 4.20) *installed on thin-walled open-topped tube. Central metal cannula is connected to a buret containing Maxidens™ via a peristaltic pump (P). Flow of Maxidens' displaces the gradient upwards into the hollow cone of the unloader. The 'O'-ring (*Figure 4.20) *directs the gradient into the side arm for collection.*

Technical variations

Collect from the top, but introduce the dense medium to the bottom of the tube by tube puncture. This mode is also feasible for sealed tubes that employ some form of central plastic plug (Chapter 2) which can be removed to leave a small neck which can simply be fitted with a delivery tube and sleeve. In practice, the Sorvall Re-Seal™ tube is the best tube type for use in this mode because the pronounced conical shoulder makes for ideal collection.

An alternative collection device which allows more flexible sampling of the gradient by upward displacement is marketed by Axis-Shield, Oslo. A rubber gasket is lowered to seal the top of the centrifuge tube. Through the gasket passes a central metal tube which is inserted to the bottom of the gradient to deliver the dense unloading solution. Around this delivery tube is a second concentric tube which can be positioned independently and it is into the annulus formed between the two tubes that the gradient is displaced and directed to the side arm (*Figure 4.22*). If the outer tube is positioned at the top of the gradient then the entire tube is unloaded; alternatively, it can be positioned at any point in the gradient to collect only that part of gradient below the annular channel.

This device was designed for use with an open-topped tubes but can also be used with some sealed tubes which use a central plastic plug.

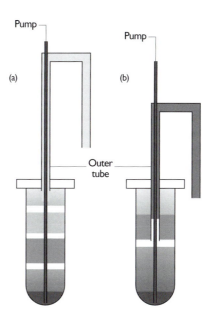

Figure 4.22

Axis-Shield upward displacement gradient unloader. (a) Collection of entire gradient: center tube delivers dense liquid to bottom of tube from pump; outer tube positioned at top of gradient. Gradient exits into annulus between the two tubes. (b) Collection of part of gradient: outer tube positioned as required.

6.5   Tube slicing

For the collection of specific zones or 'cuts' of a gradient, a tube slicer may
be a useful alternative (*Figure 4.23*). It can only be used with thin-walled
tubes and its most common use is to remove material banded close to the
top of a gradient (e.g. plasma lipoproteins floated on a density barrier). The
tube is held vertically within the tube slicer by two silicone rubber rings and
its position adjusted so that when the knife blade is advanced between the
rings, the liquid above the knife blade is isolated from the rest of the gradient (the rings providing an effective seal at the cut). The medium above the
blade can be recovered completely and the walls of the tube washed to
remove any material adhering to them.

Once the top 'cut' has been aspirated, it is feasible to withdraw the knife,
raise the tube within the slicer and make another cut to isolate an adjacent
zone of the gradient, but this is practically difficult to achieve without dis-
turbing the gradient below the first cut.

6.6   Automatic aspiration from the meniscus

The Auto Densi-flow™ which is produced by the Labconco Corporation
comprises a hollow metal tube which terminates in a small collection head
(*Figure 4.24*); the upper end of the tube is connected to a peristaltic pump
which aspirates the gradient. A motor advances the collection head towards
the gradient until the tip of an electronic probe, which is mounted at the
side of the collection head, detects the meniscus of the gradient. As the
motor is activated whenever the probe is not in contact with the meniscus,
aspiration of the gradient and the consequent fall of the meniscus will cause
the motor to advance the collection head continuously. In this way, the
entire gradient is collected in a smooth and continuous fashion. It can be
used with virtually any tube which allows access to the top and can be successfully used with tube volumes as low as 3 ml.

■   This device can also be used in a 'reversed' mode to deposit a gradient
in a tube from a two-chamber gradient maker, dense end first.

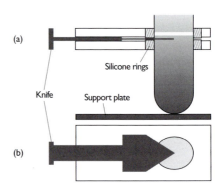

Figure 4.23

*Tube slicer: side view (a), plan view (b). Tube rests on support plate, within two silicone rings;
the knife is advanced between the two silicone rings to cut the tube so the band above the knife
cut is isolated and may be aspirated completely.*

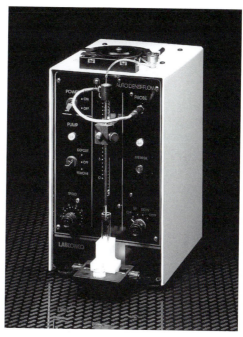

Figure 4.24

Labconco Auto Densi-flow gradient collector. For details see text. Reproduced with kind permission of Labconco Corp., Kansas City, MO, USA.

In the Brandel Microfractionator™, an 'O' ring around a metal cylinder makes a watertight seal with the tube wall and as a stepper motor advances the cylinder into the tube the gradient is forced up through the central channel. The disadvantage over the Auto Densi-flow™ is that a separate metal cylinder is required for each tube size and it is restricted to open-topped tubes. On the plus side, it is the only machine known to the author which can deal with a gradient volume as low as 0.2 ml. Moreover, each small column of liquid which is forced upwards by each advance of the cylinder enters a T-piece to be expelled into the collecting tubes by an air column (in the manner of an autoanalyzer). Thus there is essentially no mixing of adjacent zones of the gradient.

References

Dobrota, M. and Hinton, R. (1992) Conditions for density gradient separations. In: *Preparative Centrifugation – A Practical Approach* (ed. D. Rickwood). IRL Press at Oxford University Press, Oxford, pp. 77–142.

Draye, J.-P., Courtoy, P.J., Quintart, J. and Baudhuin, P. (1987) Relations between plasma membrane and lysosomal membrane. 2. Quantitative evaluation of plasma membrane marker enzymes in the lysosomes. *Eur. J. Biochem.*, **170:** 405–411.

Hames, B.D. (1984) Choice of conditions for density gradient centrifugation. In: *Centrifugation – A Practical Approach* (ed. D. Rickwood). IRL Press at Oxford University Press, Oxford, pp. 45–93.

Rickwood, D. (1992) Centrifugal methods for characterizing macromolecules and their interactions. In: *Preparative Centrifugation – A Practical Approach* (ed. D. Rickwood). IRL Press at Oxford University Press, Oxford, pp. 143–186.

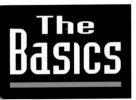

Chapter 5

Purification of mammalian cells

1. Introduction

The use of density gradients to fractionate different types of mammalian cell has been well covered in a companion volume in this series (Patel, 2001a) and to avoid large-scale repetition of both the background theory and protocols, this chapter will concentrate on some recent advances in isolation of low-density cell populations by flotation from a dense load zone through density barriers or discontinuous gradients or more simply by adjusting the mixed cell suspension to an appropriate density (i.e. the sample itself acts as the density barrier). Most of the protocols are new and are taken from recently published papers, but a few will update one or two of those which have already been described in Patel (2001a).

2. Selection of medium

Retention of maximum viability and function of cells during (and after) purification by gradient centrifugation poses one of the biggest separation problems in cell biology. The environment of the cells in the gradient should be as close as possible to that of the *in vivo* or culture situation. Choice of a medium is therefore probably more critical for cells than for any other particle. The medium should be inert and nontoxic to the cells and be able to maintain an osmolality close to that of the cells throughout the gradient, so that the cells neither gain nor lose water. Osmotic stress of cells seriously affects their density and viability (which is not easily reversed) and differences in density between cell types is often very much smaller than that between different types of organelle and membrane vesicle. Thus, sucrose, which found such an easy and wide applicability for the fractionation of subcellular organelles, is totally unsuitable for mammalian cells; indeed sucrose is considered toxic to most cells. Although some of the other polyhydric alcohols such as glycerol and mannitol are much less toxic, the high osmolality of their solutions also restricts their use for the fractionation of cells. While Ficoll™ or dextran solutions offer massive reductions in osmolality, their high viscosity and the tendency of these polysaccharides to adhere to cell surfaces makes them less than ideal. Nevertheless, there are a few important applications that have been developed using these polymers; gradients of arabinogalactan (a polysaccharide from plant sources), for example, are quite widely used for the enrichment of reticulocytes from erythrocyte fractions of human peripheral blood (e.g. Waugh, 1991).

Significant development of techniques for the fractionation of cells therefore only became possible with the introduction of the iodinated density gradient media and Percoll®. These media are generally nontoxic to mammalian cells and offer gradients that are isoosmotic. The earlier ionic forms of the iodinated density gradient media are today principally used for the commercial human lymphocyte (e.g. Lymphoprep® and Ficoll Hypaque®) and polymorphonuclear leukocyte (e.g. Polymorphprep®) isolation media (see Section 5). The majority of published methods for the separation of other blood cells types and other nonblood cells tend to use a nonionic medium such as Nycodenz® or iodixanol.

It is worth pointing out, however, that since the iodinated density gradient media were originally developed as X-ray imaging agents, only Nycodenz® and iodixanol have been exhaustively tested clinically for possible adverse effects on cells (Mützel and Speck, 1980; Nossen et al., 1990; Salvesen, 1980). The endotoxin levels in these media are accordingly very low (<0.1 EU ml^{-1}), while for Percoll® the values are <6.0 EU ml^{-1}. There is also evidence that the colloidal silica particles of Percoll® can be engulfed by phagocytic cells (Wakefield et al., 1982). The small amounts of free PRT present in Percoll® may also be detrimental to some cells

An advantage of using Percoll® for cells is that, since it has no intrinsic osmotic activity itself, the gradient media that are prepared from it (Section 3.1 and Chapter 1), can contain all of the components present in standard cell culture and suspension media at their normal concentrations. This is not possible with other media which are true solutes and which have a finite osmolality.

Occasionally a medium will be chosen with a deliberately raised or lowered osmolality to alter the buoyant density of a particular cell type selectively in order to enhance the separation of cells whose densities are very similar. This strategy has been used for human monocytes (Section 6) and it also aids the separation of acinar cells from Islets of Langerhans from disaggregated pancreas (Section 8).

3.   Handling of gradient media

The general manner in which isoosmotic gradient solutions are prepared from Percoll®, Nycodenz® and OptiPrep™ using buffered salt media (and other media containing glucose, etc.) are described in Patel (2001a). An important consideration in flotation separations is that the sample must be adjusted to an appropriately high density by addition of a dense medium. In the case of Percoll®, the commercial solution must be made isoosmotic first (Percoll® itself has essentially zero osmolality). On the other hand, when OptiPrep™ is added to an isoosmotic cell suspension medium, the osmolality will remain essentially unaltered, particularly if the added volume is small (less than 25% of the cell suspension). This simple approach may be quite satisfactory for some cell types (e.g. the preparation of mononuclear cells from whole blood).

The complete retention of cell viability and normal cell function, however, often requires a more rigorous attention to the in vitro environment. Some cell types that may be rather sensitive to gradient composition and the 'assaults' of operational handling might be better preserved if the gradient media more closely resemble culture media and if the number of centrifugation steps is kept to a minimum. Monocytes, for example, are easily activated by repeated centrifugation and resuspension and their microscopical appearance and functional viability is enhanced if solutions used for addition to the cell suspension and for density gradient layers are prepared by initial dilution of OptiPrep™ or Percoll® with a culture medium containing serum.

3.1 Preparation of gradient solutions containing culture medium and serum

Stock working solutions of OptiPrep™ and Percoll® containing culture medium and serum can be produced in a number of ways and their density and the density of gradient solutions prepared from them will be marginally higher than those produced using for example a Hepes-buffered saline (*Table 5.1*) and will depend on the final concentration of serum.

OptiPrep™ working solutions

It is not necessary that the concentration of serum in the gradient solutions is the same as that used normally for cell culture (10%, v/v); lower concentrations will suffice. For example, a simple 40% (w/v) iodixanol working solution can be made by diluting 4 volumes of OptiPrep™ with 2 volumes of Roswell Park Memorial Institute (RPMI) medium (or Dulbecco's modified Eagle's medium; DMEM) containing 10% (v/v) serum. This can be used to raise the density of a cell suspension and gradient solutions made by further dilution with the same serum-containing medium (*Table 5.1*).

If maintenance of the routine serum concentration (10%, v/v) is important, then dilute 4 volumes of OptiPrep™ with 0.6 volumes of serum (ρ = 1.03 g ml^{-1}) and 1.4 volumes of RPMI. This strategy slightly raises the density of the higher density solutions (*Table 5.1*).

Percoll®

In the case of Percoll®, the first step must, as always, be the preparation of an isoosmotic solution, in this case by dilution of 9 volumes of Percoll® with 1 volume of a 10× concentration of RPMI or DMEM (these are widely available commercially). Once this 90% (v/v) Percoll® working solution has been

Table 5.1. Density of solutions prepared from OptiPrep™-containing RPMI + serum

WS-1 (ml)	Diluent (ml)	Density (g ml^{-1})	WS-2 (ml)	Diluent (ml)	Density (g ml^{-1})
10	0	1.216	10	0	1.217
9	1	1.195	9	1	1.196
8	2	1.175	8	2	1.176
7	3	1.154	7	3	1.155
6	4	1.133	6	4	1.134
5	5	1.113	5	5	1.113
4	6	1.092	4	6	1.092
3	7	1.071	3	7	1.071
2	8	1.050	2	8	1.050
1	9	1.030	1	9	1.030

WS-1, 4 vol OptiPrep™ + 2 vol RPMI containing 10% serum; WS-2, 4 vol OptiPrep™ + 0.6 vol serum + 1.4 ml RPMI; diluent = RPMI containing 10% serum.

produced (which will have the same density as any similar salt-based isoosmotic stock) it is diluted a second time by adding serum to 10% (v/v). This
solution will have a density of 1.113 g ml^{-1} and is then further diluted with
culture medium-containing serum as required (*Table 5.2*).

Hyperosmotic solutions

Occasionally modulation of the osmolality of the suspending solution
and/or density barrier can beneficially and selectively raise the density of
one (or more) of the cell types.

Any Nycodenz® solution above $\rho = 1.15$ g ml^{-1} is hyperosmotic (see
Chapter 3) and use of NycoPrep™ Universal, which is a commercially produced solution of 60% (w/v) Nycodenz® with an osmolality of 595 mOsm
can be added to a cell suspension or diluted with any suitable solution.
Because both OptiPrep™ and Percoll® have a low osmolality (see Chapter 3),
these must be diluted with solutions of a correspondingly higher osmolality. The equation (see Chapter 3) which permits the calculation of the
density achieved by the mixing of two solutions can also be used to calculate, approximately, the osmolality of the final solution, but accurate values
can only be obtained experimentally with an osmometer. There are a
number of such devices available commercially and the most common ones
use depression of freezing point as the mode of measurement.

■   Note that the use of hyperosmotic media will also increase the density
     of the solutions produced from them compared to those produced by
     similar isoosmotic media.

4. Centrifugation strategy

Flotation of particles through a gradient often avoids some of the problems
that are inherent in sedimentation (see Chapter 1). This approach has particular relevance to the isolation of leukocytes from whole blood and to the
fractionation of tissue digests. The vast preponderance of cells in whole
blood are erythrocytes which tend *in vitro* to aggregate together to form
rouleaux and tissue digests will contain aggregates of cells which might not

Table 5.2. Density solutions prepared from Percoll®-containing RPMI + serum

WS (ml)	Diluent (ml)	Density (g ml^{-1})
10		1.113
9	1	1.103
8	2	1.092
7	3	1.082
6	4	1.071
5	5	1.061
4	6	1.051
3	7	1.040
2	8	1.030
1	9	1.020

WS, 9 vol of iso-osmotic Percoll® + 1 vol of serum (see text); Diluent, RPMI containing 10%
serum.

be removed by filtration. In both of these cases the rapid sedimentation of the larger particles may trap other cells and also lead to disturbances at gradient interfaces (see Chapter 1).

Another consideration is temperature. Many cell separation protocols are carried out at room temperature, the rationale being that since cells function optimally at 37°C, separations should be carried out as close to that temperature as possible. However, since a small percentage of cells will invariably be disrupted by the handling procedures, a case could also be made for carrying out all gradient operations at 4°C to minimize the degradative effects of any released intracellular enzymes. Moreover, cells that are potentially phagocytic may start to engulf the extracellular medium, which may not only affect their functional state but also modulate their density. In instances where lytic enzymes (e.g. collagenase) have been used to disaggregate a tissue, residual amounts of these enzymes may evade the subsequent washing procedure and continue to pose a potential degradative effect on the cells. All of these processes are inhibited at 4°C (see *Protocols 5.2* and *5.4* for examples).

Because of the fragile nature of many cells, particularly after they have been subjected to degradative enzymes during tissue disaggregation procedures (Patel, 2001b), it is often preferable to band them at an interface rather than allowing them to pellet. In this way the potentially harmful shearing forces, which are needed to resuspend a pellet, are avoided. In addition, since relative centrifugal fields (RCFs) of 400–1000 g are commonly required for any gradient centrifugation, flotation to an interface towards the top of the centrifugation tube reduces the hydrostatic pressure experienced by the cells of interest. Any subsequent pelleting of the cells from the gradient (after dilution with buffer or culture medium) should be carried out at the minimum RCF required to pellet the cell (usually 200–300 g for 10–20 min is sufficient) – again reducing the potential harmful effects of the hydrostatic pressure and the severity of any subsequent shearing forces to form a suspension from the pellet.

4.1   Practical tips

Banding of cells

In any flotation protocol, never allow the cells of interest to band at the meniscus of the low-density barrier, always layer a small volume (0.5 ml is quite sufficient) of the culture medium (or other medium used to prepare the gradient solutions) on top. This practice prevents the cells from banding at an air/water interface. If this occurs, aggregation of the cells at the junction of the meniscus with the tube wall often follows.

Rotor operation

It is good practice to avoid the use of the brake during deceleration of the rotor as the Coriolis forces, which set up a swirling effect in the liquid whenever there is a sudden change in the rate of revolution of the rotor, can cause the banded cells to mix into the infranatant, making visualization of the band more difficult (particularly a problem with small numbers of cells). Use of a slow-programmed acceleration might be beneficial for the similar reasons.

Scaling-up of methods

Use of sample volumes greater than those in the protocol are often permissible, as long as the volumes of the solutions are increased proportionally. What is perhaps more important, however, is that if, for example, the protocol uses a 15 ml centrifuge tube, then in a larger centrifuge tube (e.g. 50 ml) the volumes should be arranged such that the linear distance occupied by each layer is more or less the same. In this way the geometry of the gradient with respect to the gravitational field is maintained – this is particularly important if the separation relies on rate of flotation as well as density.

■   An important aim for any cell separation is to minimize the number of operational steps and to avoid the repeated pelleting of the cells of interest.

5.   Peripheral blood mononuclear cells

Mononuclear cells from human peripheral blood are routinely separated from erythrocytes and polymorphonuclear (PMN) leukocytes (granulocytes) by centrifugation of whole diluted blood on a barrier ($\rho = 1.077$ g ml^{-1}) according to a method devised by Bøyum (1968). The barrier regularly comprises metrizoate or diatrizoate and a polysaccharide (Ficoll™ or polysucrose) and it is available commercially from several companies (Patel, 2001a). The polysaccharide causes aggregation of the erythrocytes and consequently allows them to sediment very rapidly, but it will also adhere to other cells and there is evidence that Ficoll™ affects the mitogenic stimulation of lymphocytes (Feucht *et al.*, 1980). In addition, both metrizoate and diatrizoate are impermeant ions and they may affect the Gibbs–Donnan equilibrium of inorganic ions across the plasma membrane. Nevertheless, the method is highly effective, yielding approximately 95% of the total mononuclear cells, and is probably one of the most widely performed cell separations in the world. However, to avoid these potential problems, the $\rho = 1.077$ g ml^{-1} medium can be made up from either Nycodenz® (Bøyum *et al.*, 1983) or OptiPrep™.

If it is necessary to process large numbers of blood samples, then the alternative strategy of adjusting the plasma of whole blood to a density of 1.077 g ml^{-1} so that the mononuclear cells float to the surface while the granulocytes and erythrocytes sediment during the centrifugation may be beneficial. Patel (2001a) describes a method in which an equal volume of a Nycodenz® solution ($\rho = 1.10$ g ml^{-1}) is mixed with the blood (Ford and Rickwood, 1990); an alternative in which the Nycodenz® solution is replaced by a much smaller volume of OptiPrep™ is described in *Protocol 5.1*, thus avoiding the production of large volumes of sample and maintaining the cellular environment as close to that of the *in vivo* condition as possible.

The density barrier method using either diatrizoate+polysaccharide or a solution of similar density containing Nycodenz® or iodixanol is not successful in resolving the mononuclear cells of the blood from nonhuman species. Apparently, the mononuclear cells in the blood of rats, mice and rabbits have a slightly higher density than those of humans. Although a correspondingly higher density barrier might be used, a density-modulation approach was found to be superior (Bøyum *et al.*, 1991). By using a Nycodenz® solution of a lower osmolality (265 mOsm), the density of mononuclear cells could be modulated downwards so that they can band on top of a solution of $\rho = 1.077$ g ml^{-1}.

However, the technique in which the plasma itself is adjusted to a density higher than the mononuclear cells and lower than that of granulocytes and erythrocytes appears to be effective for mouse, rat and bovine blood without recourse to osmolality manipulation (*Protocol 5.1*). The amount of OptiPrep™ required for rat blood is marginally higher than that needed for humans and the strategy adopted for mouse blood is modified to take account of the rather small volumes of sample (*Protocol 5.1*). Why the flotation mode works more satisfactorily than the density-barrier sedimentation strategy for mouse and rat blood (in the absence of osmolality modulation) is not very clear. It may reflect the tendency of the platelets in blood from these experimental animals to sediment to and aggregate at the barrier more quickly than is the case with human blood.

6. Human monocytes

The monocytes in human peripheral blood, account for, on average, about 8% of the leukocyte population. They tend to be larger (15–20 µm) than lymphocytes (6–20 µm) and they also have a slightly lower density (*Figure 5.1*). The density difference alone is insufficient to allow an effective and efficient separation and the rates of sedimentation are similar (the lower density of the monocytes being offset by their larger size). Bøyum *et al.* (1983) therefore devised a Nycodenz® barrier of density 1.068 g ml^{-1} and an osmolality of 335 mOsm in order to separate monocytes and lymphocytes from human peripheral blood. Because lymphocytes are more sensitive the osmotic pressure of the suspending solution, these cells lose water more rapidly than do monocytes and consequently the density difference between the two cell types is enhanced.

Although sedimentation rates of the two types of cell are similar (in their native state), both the larger size and lower density of monocytes contribute to a more rapid rate of flotation. If the density of a leukocyte-rich plasma is raised to ~ 1.13 g ml^{-1}, the leukocytes will float to the top of the plasma (*Figure 5.2*) when this suspension is centrifuged. In this way, the mononuclear

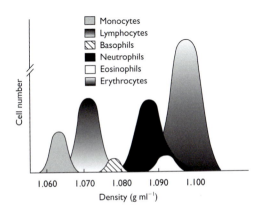

Figure 5.1

Density of human blood cells.

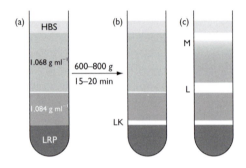

Figure 5.2

Isolation of human monocytes by flotation from a leukocyte-rich plasma (LRP). (a) The LRP is adjusted to a density of approximately 1.13 g ml⁻¹ and layered beneath two iodixanol layers and Hepes-buffered saline (HBS). (b) During centrifugation the leukocytes (LK) rapidly float to the top of the load zone. (c) From the LK layer the monocytes (M) float to the top of the gradient more rapidly than the lymphocytes (L).

cells rapidly form a narrow band at the interface between the sample and a 1.084-g ml⁻¹ solution layered on top. The monocytes (because of their size and density) migrate upwards through this layer and through a second low-density barrier (ρ = 1.068 g ml⁻¹). The smaller and denser lymphocytes tend to float more slowly, and in this way a separation between the two types of cells is effected (Graziani-Bowering *et al.*, 1997).

   Yields of cells are variable (10–40%) which may reflect (i) the requirement to produce a leukocyte-rich plasma (LRP) first; (ii) the use of non-optimal solutions for density enhancement of the LRP and (iii) the use of room temperature for the centrifugation (Section 4).

   The method has recently been modified in a manner that redresses these operational problems, that is, a single centrifugation is used; gradient solutions contain culture medium and serum, and centrifugation is carried out at 4°C (*Protocol 5.2*). A single low-density barrier is placed on top of whole blood; the density of the barrier may be 1.072 or 1.074 g ml⁻¹ (*Figure 5.3*). The lower density barrier yields a more pure monocyte fraction (approximatley 90% vs. 80–85%) but the yields are lower (40% vs. 60%).

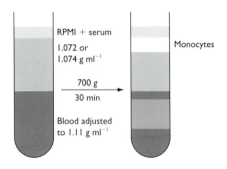

Figure 5.3

Isolation of human monocytes by flotation from whole blood.

7.   Dendritic cells

Since dendritic cells (DC) were recognized as playing an important role in the induction of cell-mediated responses (Barfoot *et al.*, 1989), there has been a rapid growth in research into the function of these cells and methods for their purification. Gradients of either albumin or metrizamide, although providing an effective enrichment of DC, tended to cause some functional alteration of the cells (McLellan *et al.*, 1995). Because cells are much more tolerant of Nycodenz®, this iodinated density-gradient medium rapidly became established as the medium of choice for DC cell purification from peripheral blood.

As DC have a relatively low density, some methods used NycoPrep™ 1.068, the ready-made solution of 13% (w/v) Nycodenz® ($\rho = 1.068$ g ml^{-1}) which was designed primarily for the isolation of monocytes from human peripheral blood (Mannering *et al.*, 1998; McLellan *et al.*, 1995). Other methods used Nycodenz® solutions (in the range 13–14.5%, w/v) usually made up in a culture medium containing serum (Van Vugt *et al.*, 1991).

New methods have been developed for isolation of DC by flotation in OptiPrep™ gradients (e.g. Ruedl *et al.*, 1996). DC have been isolated from a variety of tissue types including peripheral blood, peripheral lymph, lymph nodes, spleen, Peyer's patches and thymus, using density barriers of 1.055–1.065 g ml^{-1} and both of the flotation strategies of adjusting the mixed cell population to the required low density, or layering the mixed cell population in a denser medium below a low-density barrier, have been used (*Protocol 5.3*).

8.   Isolation of Islets of Langerhans from porcine pancreas

This is an example of the use of a flotation technique to isolate a low-density population of cells from a tissue digest. It also provides an example of the use of a hyperosmotic medium in order to enhance the difference in density between acinar cells (the denser cell type) from the Islets. This has also been chosen because it illustrates the use of a density gradient in an application, which has both clinical and commercial implications in the treatment of diabetes, by the use of implants of Islets. The Islets must not only function properly, they must also not be contaminated by the acinar cells that are the source of degradative proteases. Moreover, the gradient medium that is used must be compatible with the potential use of the gradient product in human transplantation.

The method that is described in *Protocol 5.4* uses OptiPrep™ gradients and emphasizes the strategy of the centrifugation rather than the precise composition of the media that are currently used. Choice of the medium that is used to dilute the OptiPrep™ will vary from laboratory to laboratory and is to some extent species-specific. For porcine pancreas, the so-called 'University of Wisconsin Solution (UWS)' has been used by Van der Burg *et al.* (1998a, b); this complex solution has been formulated specifically for porcine pancreas.

To raise the density of the digest suspension (in UWS) to $\rho = 1.10$ g ml^{-1}, it is mixed with half of its volume of a 30% (w/v) iodixanol working solution. A low-density barrier ($\rho = 1.09$ g ml^{-1}) is similarly produced by mixing the working solution with UWS. This working solution is prepared by mixing OptiPrep™ (60% iodixanol) with an equal volume of 2× UWS. UWS itself, like any cell suspension medium, is isoosmotic; by using 2× UWS, the 30% iodixanol working solution has an osmolality of approximatley 500 mOsm, thus the osmolality of both the digest suspension and the low density barrier is 370–380 mOsm.

■   Note that the use of a hyperosmotic diluent will not only raise the osmolality of the working solution, it will also raise its density (in this case to approximately 1.21 g ml^{-1}) compared to a working solution prepared from a similar isoosmotic solution.

The protocol uses a 50-ml conical centrifuge tube in which the density of the Islet suspension is raised by mixing with the working solution (WS) before a low-density barrier (ρ = 1.09 g ml^{-1}) and UWS are layered on top. During centrifugation, the Islets float to the interface between the UWS and the ρ = 1.09 g ml^{-1} barrier, while the acinar tissue remains in the load zone (*Figure 5.4*).

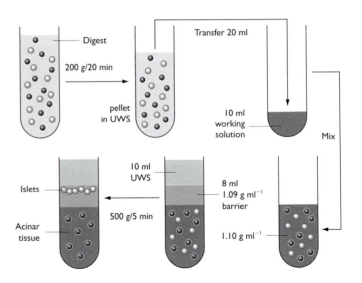

Figure 5.4

Purification of Islets of Langerhans from enzyme digests of porcine pancreas. See text for details; UWS, University of Wisconsin solution.

9. Stellate cells from mammalian liver

The fractionation of hepatic nonparenchymal (sinusoidal) cells (Kupffer cells, stellate cells, endothelial cells, etc.) on continuous metrizamide (Bøyum *et al.*, 1983) and Nycodenz® gradients (Brouwer *et al.*, 1991) has shown that the overlap in banding densities of these cells makes these gradients generally unsatisfactory as a stand-alone procedure to isolate the various cell populations. Consequently other strategies, such as the use of centrifugal elutriation are required (Patel, 2000c).

Stellate cells, however, are the least dense of the nonparenchymal cells and can be floated effectively away from the rest of the cells (*Protocol 5.5*). The low-density fraction produced may contain almost 80% stellate cells (Brouwer *et al.*, 1991); methods commonly use a barrier of 1.067 g ml^{-1} (Elsharkawy *et al.*, 1999; Trim *et al.*, 2000), but densities as low as 1.053 g ml^{-1} have been used (Cassiman *et al.*, 1999).

10. Other low-density cells

The proliferation and maturation of *hematopoietic stem cells* from bone marrow and how these processes are regulated are major areas of cell and molecular biology research. The resolving power of density gradients is, however, insufficient to allow megakaryocytic progenitor cells to be isolated in a sufficiently pure form for further analysis and culture. Nevertheless, they do provide a useful preliminary purification step that can usually achieve a two–threefold enrichment of these cells from crude bone marrow samples. This allows a more economical and effective use immunomagnetic beads to remove lineage cells using a cocktail of lineage-specific monoclonal antibodies.

The progenitor cells have a density of less than 1.08 g ml^{-1} and the appropriate density barrier can be produced by dilution of OptiPrep™ with a balanced salt solution (with or without 5% fetal calf serum; FCS) to give a 14% w/v iodixanol (Hodohara *et al.*, 2000). Although in the published method the bone marrow cell suspension was layered over the barrier and centrifuged at 450 *g* for 20 min, the flotation method may produce improved resolution.

Reticulocytes, which are the precursors of mammalian erythrocytes, tend to be less dense than the mature cells and, although the standard approach of layering a washed erythrocyte suspension on top of a gradient is the commonly employed method, this particular separation, in which the cells of interest represent such a small proportion of the total cells (from normal blood), may benefit from the flotation strategy.

References

Barfoot, R., Denham, S., Gyure, L.A., Hall, J.G., Hobbs, S.M., Jackson, L.E. and Robertson, D. (1989) Some properties of dendritic macrophages from peripheral lymph. *Immunol.* **68**: 233–239.

Bøyum, A. (1968) Isolation of mononuclear cells and granulocytes from human blood. *Scand. J. Clin. Lab. Invest.* **21** (Suppl. 97): 77–89.

Bøyum, A., Berg, T. and Blomhoff, R. (1983) Fractionation of mammalian cells. In: *Iodinated Density Gradient Media – a Practical Approach* (ed. D. Rickwood). IRL Press at Oxford University Press, Oxford, UK, pp 147–171.

Bøyum, A., Løvhaug, D., Tresland, L. and Nordlie, E.M. (1991) Separation of leucocytes: improved cell purity by fine adjustment of gradient medium density and osmolarity. *Scand. J. Immunol.* **34**: 697–712.

Brouwer, A., Hendricks, H.F.J., Ford, T. and Knook, D.L. (1991) Centrifugal separations of mammalian cells. In: *Preparative Centrifugation – a Practical Approach* (ed. D. Rickwood). IRL Press at Oxford University Press, Oxford, UK, pp 271–314.

Cassiman, D., van Pelt, J., De Vos, R., Van Lommel, F., Desmet, V., Yap, S-H. and Roskams, T. (1999) Synaptophysin: a novel marker for human and rat hepatic stellate cells. *Am. J. Pathol.* **155**: 1831–1839.

Elsharkawy, A.M., Wright, M.C., Hay, R.T., Arthur, M.J.P., Hughes, T., Bahr, M.J., Degitz, K. and Mann, D.A. (1999) Persistent activation of nuclear factor-κB in cultured rat hepatic stellate cells involves the induction of potentially novel Rel like factors and prolonged changes in the expression of IκB family protein Hepatology **30**: 761–769.

Ford, T.C. and Rickwood, D. (1990) A new one-step method for the isolation of human mononuclear cells. J. Immunol. Meth. **134**: 237–241.

Graziani-Bowering, G.M., Graham, J.M. and Filion, L.G. (1997) A quick, easy and inexpensive method for the isolation of human peripheral blood monocytes. J. Immunol. Meth. **207**: 157–168.

Hodohara, K., Fujii, N., Yamamoto, N. and Kaushansky, K. (2000) Stromal cell derived factor (SDF-1) acts together with thrombopoietin to enhance the development of megakaryocytic progenitor cells (CFU-MK). Blood, **95**: 769–775.

Mannering, S.I., McKenzie, J.L. and Hart, D.N.J. (1998) Optimisation of the conditions for generating human DC initiated antigen specific T lymphocyte lines in vitro. J. Immunol. Meth. **219**: 69–83.

McLellan, A.D., Starling, G.C. and Hart, D.N.J. (1995) Isolation of human blood dendritic cells by discontinuous Nycodnez gradient centrifugation. J. Immunol Meth. **184**: 81–89.

Nossen, J.Ø., Aakhus, T., Berg, K.J., Jørgensen, N.P. and Andrew, EW. (1990 Experience with iodixanol, a new nonionic dimeric contrast medium preliminary results from the human phase I study. Invest. Radiol. **25**: S113–S114.

Mützel, W. and Speck, U. (1980) Pharmacokinetics and biotransformation of iohexol in the rat and the dog. Acta Radiol., **362** (Suppl.): 87–92.

Patel, D. (2001a) Fractionation of cells by sedimentation methods. In: Separating Cells. BIOS Scientific Publishers Ltd, Oxford, UK, pp. 48–86.

Patel, D. (2001b) Preparation of cell suspensions. In: Separating Cells. BIOS Scientific Publishers Ltd, Oxford, UK, pp. 1–47.

Patel, D. (2001c) Centrifugal elutriation. In: Separating Cells. BIOS Scientific Publishers Ltd, Oxford, UK, pp. 87–106.

Ruedl, C., Rieser, C., Böck, G., Wick, G. and Wolf, H. (1996) Phenotypic and functional characterization of CD11c+ dendritic cell population in mouse Peyer' patches. Eur. J. Immunol., **26**: 1801–1806.

Salvesen, S. (1980). Acute intravenous toxicity of iohexol in the mouse and in the rat Acta Radiol, **362** (Suppl.): 73–75.

Trim, J.E., Samra, S.K., Arthur, M.J.P., Wright, M.C., McAulay, M., Beri, R. and Mann, D.A. (2000) Upstream tissue inhibitor of metalloproteinases-1 (TIMP-1 element-1, a novel and essential regulatory motif in the human TIMP-1 gene promoter, directly interacts with a 30-kDa nuclear protein. J. Biol. Chem. **275** 6657–6663.

Van der Burg, M.P.M., Basir, I., Zwaan, R.P. and Bouwman, E. (1998a) Porcine islet preservation during isolation in University of Wisconsin solutions Transplant Proc. **30**: 360–361.

Van der Burg, M.P.M., Basir, I. and Bouwman, E. (1998b) No porcine loss during density gradient purification in a novel iodixanol/University of Wisconsin solution. Transplant. Proc. **30**: 362–363.

Van Vugt, E., Arkema, J.M.S., Verdaasdonk, M.A.M., Beelen, R.H.J. and Kamperdijk E.W.A. (1991) Morphological and functional characteristics of rat steady state peritoneal dendritic cells. Immunobiol. **184**: 14–24.

Wakefield, J. StJ., Gale, J.S., Berridge, M.V., Jordan, T.W. and Ford, H.C. (1982) Is Percoll innocuous to cells? Biochem. J. **202**: 795–797.

Waugh., R.E. (1991) Reticulocyte rigidity and passage through endothelial-like pores Blood **78**: 3037–3042.

Protocol 5.1

Purification of mononuclear cells by flotation from whole blood (human, rat and mouse)

Equipment

Low-speed centrifuge with swinging-bucket rotor to accommodate 15-ml tubes

Syringe for collecting blood (size varies with blood volume).

Reagents

OptiPrep™

Tricine-buffered saline (TBS, mouse blood only): 0.85% (w/v) NaCl, 10 mM Tricine–NaOH, pH 7.4.

Protocol

Sample collection

1. Collect human peripheral blood by standard venepuncture using EDTA (1 mM) or citrate (3.8%, w/v) as anticoagulant (heparin should be avoided for best results).

2. Collect rat blood by anesthetizing the animal with CO_2 and collect blood ($\sim$10 ml from an adult male rat) into a 10 ml syringe containing 1 ml of 3.8% (w/v) citrate.

3. Collect mouse by anesthetizing the animal with CO_2 and collect blood (0.5–1.0 ml) into a 2 ml syringe containing 0.1 ml of 3.8% (w/v) citrate.

Fractionation of cells

1. Mix well 1.25 ml (for human blood) or 1.26 ml (for rat blood) of OptiPrep™ with 10 ml of blood by gentle, repeated inversion. For mouse blood (0.5–1.0 ml) mix 5.0 ml of TBS with 1.5 ml of OptiPrep™ and then mix gently 5 ml of this solution with the blood.

2. Layer a small volume ($\sim$0.5 ml) of saline on top. This avoids the mononuclear cells banding at an air/water interface and also the tendency for the cells to pile up at the plasma/tube wall junction.

3. Centrifuge at 1000–1200 g_{av} for 30 min at 20°C.

4. Collect the cells using a Pasteur pipette placed at the meniscus, removing all of the supernatant down to about 2 cm from the pellet.

Notes

Most of the cells will band at the plasma/saline interface but 10–15% will be in the plasma phase above the pellet.

Protocol 5.2

Purification of monocytes by flotation from whole human blood

Equipment

Low-speed centrifuge with swinging-bucket rotor to accommodate 15 ml tubes (set to 4°C).

Syringe for collecting blood (size varies with blood volume).

Reagents

OptiPrep™

Diluent: standard culture medium (RPMI or DMEM) containing 10% (v/v) serum.

Protocol

1. Prepare a 40% (w/v) iodixanol WS by diluting 4 volumes of OptiPrep™ with 2 vol of diluent. This has a density of approximately 1.216 g ml^{-1}.

2. Collect human peripheral blood by standard venepuncture using EDTA (1 mM) as anticoagulant.

3. Bring blood, all solutions and centrifuge tubes to 4°C.

4. Prepare *either* a 1.072-g ml^{-1} *or* a 1.074-g ml^{-1} density-barrier solution by diluting WS with diluent: 2.14 ml + 5 ml or 2.27 + 5 ml respectively.

5. Mix 4.24 ml of WS with 10 ml of whole blood; do this by repeated but gentle inversion.

6. In a 15 ml centrifuge tube, layer 5 ml of one of the density-barrier solutions over 5 ml of the blood, and then layer approximatley 0.5 ml of diluent on top.

7. Centrifuge at 700 g in a swinging-bucket rotor for 30 min at 4°C. Do not use the brake during deceleration.

8. Collect the monocytes that float to the top of the 1.072- or 1.074-g ml^{-1} layer.

9. Dilute the collected cells with 2 volumes of diluent and harvest by centrifugation at 200–300 g for 20 min. Then resuspend the pellet gently in any medium as required.

Notes

This strategy has been adapted to rat blood, using 1.074–1.076-g ml^{-1} density barriers. There are proportionately fewer monocytes in rat blood than in human blood and to achieve an adequate yield it may be necessary to sacrifice purity.

Protocol 5.3

Purification of dendritic cells by flotation from mouse tissues (Ruedl *et al.*, 1996)

The protocol for dissociating the tissue will vary with the type of tissue and is beyond the scope of this text. For more information see Patel (2001b) and Ruedl *et al.* (1996).

Equipment

Low-speed centrifuge with swinging-bucket rotor to accommodate 15 ml tubes (set to 4°C).

Reagents

Filtered tissue digest

OptiPrep™

Cell suspension solution (CSS): Hank's balanced salt solution (without Ca^{2+} and Mg^{2+})

Diluent: 0.88% (w/v) NaCl, 1 mM EDTA, 0.5% (w/v) bovine serum albumin, 10 mM Hepes–NaOH, pH 7.4.

Protocol

1. Make up an 11.5% (w/v) iodixanol solution ($\rho = 1.065$ g ml^{-1}) from OptiPrep™ and the diluent (1:4.2 v/v).

2. Harvest the cells from the filtered tissue digest by centrifugation and wash them as required in a balanced salt medium.

3. Suspend the washed cell pellet in CSS.

4. Mix gently but thoroughly with OptiPrep™ (3:1 v/v) to give a 15% (w/v) iodixanol solution ($\rho = 1.085$ g ml^{-1}).

5. Overlayer 4 ml of this suspension with 5 ml of 11.5% iodixanol and 3 ml of CSS.

6. Centrifuge at 600 g_{av} for 15 min at approximately 20°C.

7. Allow the rotor to decelerate without the brake and harvest the DC from the top of the 11.5% iodixanol layer.

Notes

It is often necessary to omit divalent cations from balanced salt media as both Mg^{2+} and Ca^{2+} can cause aggregation of cells at interfaces.

Protocol 5.4

Purification of Islets of Langerhans by flotation from digested porcine pancreas (Van der Burg *et al.* 1998a, b)

The protocol for dissociating the tissue and the optimal composition of the Islet suspension medium will vary from laboratory to laboratory (it will also vary with the species used). These matters are beyond the scope of this text, which is aimed principally at the isolation strategy. For more information see Van der Burg *et al.* (1998a, b) and Patel (2001b).

Equipment

Low-speed centrifuge with swinging-bucket rotor to accommodate 50 ml tubes (set to 4°C).

Reagents

OptiPrep™

Diluent A: Islet suspension medium at 2× normal concentration (e.g. 2× UWS).

Diluent B: for gradient solutions: e.g. UWS.

Protocol

1. Keep all solutions and carry out all operations at 4°C.

2. Prepare the WS ($\rho = 1.206$ g ml^{-1}): mix equal volumes of OptiPrep™ and Diluent A.

3. Transfer 10 ml aliquots of the WS to 50 ml conical centrifuge tubes.

4. Prepare the low-density barrier solution ($\rho = 1.090$ g ml^{-1}): mix 10 ml WS with 26.36 ml of UWS.

5. Centrifuge the digest for 2 min at 200 g and gently resuspend the pellet in UWS (for a 10 ml cell pellet make up to 80 ml).

6. Transfer 20 ml of suspension into each of the prepared centrifuge tubes containing 10 ml of WS and mix rapidly but gently by repeated inversion.

7. Layer 8 ml of the low-density barrier solution over the suspension and top up the tube with 10 ml of UWS.

8. Centrifuge at 500 g for 5 min at 4°C. The Islets band at the top interface; acinar tissue remains in the load zone.

9. Harvest the islets using a syringe and wide-bore metal cannula; dilute with an equal volume of UWS and pellet at 200 g for 4 min.

Protocol 5.5

Purification of stellate cells from mammalian liver

The protocol for dissociating the tissue will vary from laboratory to laboratory (it will also vary with the species used). These matters are beyond the scope of this text, which is aimed principally at the isolation strategy. For more information see Brouwer et al. (1991) and Patel (2001b).

Equipment

Low-speed centrifuge with swinging-bucket rotor to accommodate 15 ml tubes (set to 4°C).

Reagents

Gey's balanced salt solution (GBSS): 7.0 g NaCl, 0.37 g KCl, 70 mg $MgSO_4 \cdot 7H_2O$, 150 mg $NaHPO_4 \cdot 2H_2O$, 220 mg $CaCl_2 \cdot 2H_2O$, 2.27 g $NaHCO_3$, 30 mg KH_2PO_4, 210 mg $MgCl_2 \cdot 6H_2O$, 1.0 g glucose dissolved in 1 liter of water, gassed with 5% CO_2/air. The pH should be 7.4.

OptiPrep™ (60% w/v, iodixanol).

Protocol

1. Suspend the crude nonparenchymal cells in GBSS ($1-4 \times 10^8$ cells).

2. Make a 40% (w/v) iodixanol WS: mix 4 volumes of OptiPrep™ and 2 volumes of GBSS.

3. Add WS to the cell suspension so that the final concentration of iodixanol is 17% (w/v) iodixanol solution ($\rho = 1.096$ g ml^{-1}).

4. Mix thoroughly but gently by repeated inversion.

5. Dilute WS with GBSS to produce a solution containing 11.5% (w/v) iodixanol.

6. Layer 5 ml of this solution over the same volume of cell suspension, then layer 2 ml of GBSS on top.

7. Centrifuge at 1400 g for 17 min.

8. Allow the rotor to decelerate without the brake.

9. Collect the cells, which band at the interface between the GBSS and the 11.5% iodixanol.

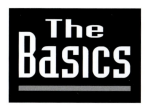

Chapter 6

Fractionation of sub-cellular organelles

Although Sections 4–5 of this chapter will describe the behavior of all sub-cellular particles during differential centrifugation of an homogenate, the density gradient systems (Section 6) will address exclusively the purification of the larger organelles which are recovered in the nuclear, heavy mitochondrial and light mitochondrial pellets. The fractionation of membrane vesicles in gradients is considered in Chapter 7.

The ability to carry out the purification of subcellular particles also relies on the ability to homogenize the chosen tissue or cells efficiently and effectively without causing significant damage to the particles. This will be briefly considered in Section 2.

1. Introduction

Many of the basic techniques of preparative centrifugation, as they are applied to the fractionation of the major subcellular organelles from rat liver, were worked out in the 1950s and 1960s by a number of research groups in Europe and the USA and pre-eminent among these groups were Christian de Duve's group working in Belgium and George Palade's group in the USA. The development of centrifugal separation techniques was achieved in concert with advances in other important areas of research technology. Validation of the efficacy of a separative technique relied on the ability to detect and identify organelles and this was made possible through important advances in the design of reliable enzyme assays and by the development of electron microscopy. These events were paralleled by important advances in the availability of reliable commercial centrifuges and the techniques used to homogenize mammalian tissue, which are covered in the next section.

2. Homogenization of tissue or cells

2.1 Aims of the homogenization procedure

The principal aim must be to achieve, reproducibly, the highest degree of cell breakage using the minimum of disruptive forces, but at the same time cause no damage to any of the organelles of interest and to avoid protein denaturation. A target cell lysis of at least 90% is generally acceptable. An obvious requirement of homogenization is to maintain, as far as is feasible, the functional integrity of the subcellular components. The homogenization procedure is the first of many of the assaults which are made on the cell and its contents: it should be recognized that as soon as the cell is broken, the environment of all its components is changed drastically so as to facilitate the subsequent fractionation steps. It would therefore be surprising if the functional competence of organelles *in vitro* were identical to that *in vivo*.

2.2   General technical problems

Functional integrity of subcellular components is compromised by foaming: this can lead to protein denaturation and it is a particular problem with mechanical shear methods. The foaming that occurs with nitrogen cavitation, although posing a handling problem, is less deleterious because the bubbles are of an inert gas rather than air.

A major problem is the redistribution of macromolecules that occurs from the cytoplasmic surface of membranes and organelles to the soluble cytosol fraction or to other organelles. Immunohistochemistry studies have shown that the type III isoenzyme of hexokinase, which is clearly localized to the nuclear periphery in kidney and liver, is found in the soluble fraction of homogenates of these tissues (Preller and Wilson, 1992). A similar problem exists with DNA polymerase, which may be found in the cytosol after release from damaged nuclei. Moreover, any protein in the soluble fraction, whether native or dissociated from the surface of an organelle during the homogenization procedure can be trapped adventitiously by vesicles formed during the process.

Release of DNA from nuclei and hydrolases from lysosomes can have serious consequences for any subsequent fractionation. Any DNA tends to adhere to other particles. Not only does this cause aggregation of these particles, it also compromises studies of the DNA in mitochondria or chloroplasts.

2.3   Liquid-shear homogenization

Potter–Elvehjem (Teflon-and-glass) homogenizer

This consists of a glass containing vessel and a pestle of machined Teflon, which is normally attached to an overhead electrical motor (*Figure 6.1*). Typically, the pestle is rotated at 500–1000 r.p.m.

■   Homogenizers with a clearance of approximately 0.09 mm are used principally for soft mammalian tissue or hard tissue (muscle) that has been enzymically 'softened'.

The Dounce (all-glass) homogenizer

The pestle is a hand-operated glass ball (*Figure 6.1*), although some small-volume variants have a ground glass cylinder. They have variable clearances but generally fall into two types:

■   loose-fitting (clearance is 0.1–0.3 mm), used mainly for soft mammalian tissue;
■   tight-fitting (clearance of 0.05–0.08 mm), used mainly for cultured cells, spheroplasts and protoplasts.

Cell cracker (ball-bearing homogenizer).

It comprises a precision bore (1.270 cm) in a stainless steel block, containing a 1.267 cm stainless steel ball. Using a system of syringes, the cell sus-

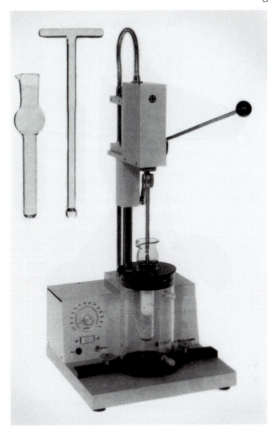

Figure 6.1

An automated version of a Potter–Elvehjem homogenizer. The Potter–Elvehjem (Teflon/glass) homogenizer is surrounded by a jacket through which cold water can be circulated. The speed of rotation of the pestle is controlled by the dial on the left and the pestle is advanced using the pivoted arm (right). The all glass Dounce homogenizer (inset top-left) is manually oper- ated. Reproduced from W.H. Evans (1992), Isolation and characterization of membranes and cell organelles. In: Preparative Centrifugation – A Practical Approach *(ed D. Rickwood). IRL Press at Oxford University Press, Oxford. With permission of Oxford University Press.*

pension can be forced repeatedly through the gap around the ball. For most cells 10–12 passes are sufficient (Balch *et al.*, 1984).

■   This is generally regarded as one of the most effective yet gentle methods for disrupting cultured cells.

Other devices

Repeated passage of the cell suspension through a narrow gage syringe needle can be a simple but effective strategy. An alternative is to force the cell suspension from a syringe through a metal screen (pore size 100 µm) or in the case of plant protoplasts through a nylon mesh of pore size 20 µm.

2.4 Mechanical shear

Mechanical shear homogenizers use rotating metal blades or teeth to disrupt the material and are always used in a pulsed mode to avoid foaming.

The Polytron homogenizer

The Polytron homogenizer (*Figure 6.2*) is by far the most commonly used form of rotating blade homogenizer. It has interchangeable workheads of different diameters for use with different volumes (down to 1–2 ml). The speed of rotation of the blades can normally be varied over a wide range (usually 2000–4000 r.p.m.).

■   It is mainly used for hard and soft mammalian tissues and plant tissues.

2.5   Nitrogen cavitation

This is used exclusively for single cell suspensions. It comprises a robust stainless steel pressure vessel with an inlet port for delivery of the gas from a cylinder and an outlet tube with a needle valve (*Figure 6.3*). A stirred cell suspension is equilibrated with oxygen-free nitrogen at pressures of about 5500 kPa (800 psi) for between 10 and 30 min. Nitrogen dissolves in the suspending medium and in the cytosol of the cells. When the needle valve is opened, the suspension is forced through the outlet tube and, as it

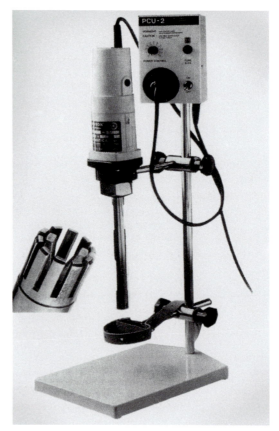

Figure 6.2

A Polytron rotating blades homogenizer. The inset shows the working head. Reproduced from W.H. Evans (1992), Isolation and characterization of membranes and cell organelles. In: Preparative Centrifigation – A Practical Approach (*eds D. Rickwood). IRL Press at Oxford University Press, Oxford. With permission of Oxford University Press.*

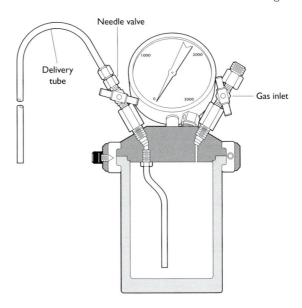

Figure 6.3

A nitrogen cavitation vessel. The cell suspension is placed in the stainless steel container and the gas-tight lid secured. The lid contains a pressure gage, an inlet for the nitrogen gas and a delivery tube. After equilibration (normally 15–20 min at 4°C) the needle valve is opened; when the cell suspension passes the valve it is exposed to atmospheric pressure and the cells are disrupted by the rapid expansion of the dissolved nitrogen. Reproduced from W.H. Evans (1992), Isolation and characterization of membranes and cell organelles. In: Preparative Centrifugation – a Practical Approach (ed D. Rickwood) IRL Press at Oxford University Press. With Permission of Oxford University Press.

becomes exposed to atmospheric pressure beyond the needle valve, it experiences a rapid decompression. Cell disruption occurs due to the sudden formation of bubbles of nitrogen gas in the cytosol and in the medium.

■ Although very efficient and highly reproducible, ribosomes tend to be stripped off the rough endoplasmic reticulum and the nuclei tend to be very fragile.

2.6 Homogenization media

Table 6.1 lists some of the commonly used media and their uses. The media for the isolation of plant organelles tend to be specific not only for the organelle but also the type of plant (see Whitehouse and Moore, 1993; Moore *et al.*, 1993; Graham, 1997, for more information).

Cultured cells

Although some cultured cells can be homogenized in an isoosmotic medium, it may be necessary to stress the cells osmotically by using a hypo-osmotic medium, for example 1 mM sodium bicarbonate, pH 8.0 or 10 mM Hepes–NaOH (or Tris–HCl) at pH 7–8 (see also *Table 6.1*).

It is very much a 'trial-and-error' procedure to optimize the medium for a particular cell type; inclusion of $MgCl_2$ may be beneficial to nuclear integrity. If EDTA is included, the nuclei may be fragile and prone to leak DNA, although inclusion of DNase I ($10 \, \mu g \, ml^{-1}$) can guard against aggregation due to the release of DNA.

Table 6.1. Homogenization media for mammalian tissues and cells

Composition	Tissue/cell type	Organelle
0.25 M sucrose, 1 mM EDTA, 10 mM Tris–HCl, pH 7–8.	Soft tissues, cultured cells	General purpose
0.25 M sucrose, 25 mM KCl, 5 mM MgCl$_2$, 10 mM Tris–HCl, pH 7.4	Soft tissues	Nuclei
0.25 M sucrose, 1 mM EDTA, 10 mM triethanolamine-acetic acid, pH 7.4	Cultured cell monolayers	General purpose
0.2 M mannitol, 50 mM sucrose, 1 mM EDTA, 10 mM Hepes–NaOH, pH 7.4	Soft tissues	Mitochondria
0.32 M sucrose, 1 mM EDTA, 10 mM Tris–HCl, pH 7–8.	Brain tissue	General purpose
0.1 M sucrose, 46 mM KCl, 10 mM EDTA, 100 mM Tris–HCl, pH 7–8	Skeletal muscle	Mitochondria, sarcoplasmic reticulum
15 mM KCl, 1.5 mM MgOAc, 1 mM dithiothreitol, 10 mM Hepes–KOH, pH 7.5	Suspension cells	General purpose[a]

[a] Hypoosmotic medium of Goldberg and Kornfeld (1983).

Hard tissues

To avoid lengthy periods of mechanical shear homogenization it is usual to break down the external fibrous tissue of skeletal muscle using a commercially available protease – Nagarse™ is the most common.

Yeast, fungi and plants

The presence of a thick and resilient cell wall has important consequences for homogenization. The severe mechanical shear which used to be employed with such material, and which also caused disruption of released organelles, has now been almost universally replaced by the use of enzymes to digest the wall material to release protoplasts (plants) or spheroplasts (yeast). These structures are delimited by a normal plasma membrane, which can be disrupted by liquid shear.

Zymolase™ is used for yeast (see Graham, 1997, for more information) and a combination of Cellulysin™ and Macerase™ for plant tissues (see Whitehouse and Moore, 1993; Moore *et al.*, 1993, for more information).

Protease inhibitors

To protect organelles from the potentially damaging effects of proteases, which may be released from lysosomes during homogenization, it is common to include a cocktail of protease inhibitors in the homogenization medium. A typical mixture for mammalian cells is 1 mM phenylmethylsulfonylfluoride (PMSF), 2 µg ml^{-1} each of leupeptin, antipain and aprotinin. These are normally stored as 100× concentration solutions, PMSF in ethanol (or isopropanol), leupeptin and antipain in 10% dimethyl sulfoxide and aprotinin in water.

3.   Physical characteristics of subcellular particles

The dimensions of the major subcellular organelles from a rat liver homogenate are given in *Table 6.2* and it is clear that they can be divided broadly into four classes based upon their size. The first group comprises

Table 6.2. Size and sedimenting properties of subcellular organelles

Particle	d (μm)	d^2 (μm^2)	$\rho_p - \rho_l$ (g ml^{-1})[a]
Nuclei	4–12	16–144	0.19–0.22
Plasma membrane sheets	3–20	9–400	0.12–0.17
Mitochondria	0.4–2.5	0.16–6.3	0.11–0.13
Lysosomes	0.4–0.8	0.16–0.64	0.07–0.11
Peroxisomes	0.4–0.8	0.16–0.64	0.14–0.17
Golgi tubules	1–2	1–4	0.03–0.06
Vesicles	0.05–0.4	0.0025–0.25	0.05–0.08

[a] The $\rho_p - \rho_l$ values are based on ρ_p in a sucrose gradient.

principally the nuclei that are by far the largest organelle; only sheets of plasma membrane are comparable in size. At the other end of the size spectrum is a second group which contains the huge array of small membrane vesicles, some which (endosomes and the vesicles involved in synthesis, transport and secretion) are present in the cell *in vivo*, while others are derived from the endoplasmic reticulum, plasma membrane and Golgi apparatus during the process of homogenization (see Chapter 7). In between is a third group comprising the major organelles, mitochondria, lysosomes and peroxisomes. Most of these are in the range 0.4–0.8 μm in diameter; however, a large proportion of the mitochondria are significantly larger (up to 2.0 μm) and the largest mitochondria form the fourth group. This group of mitochondria also tends to be denser and they are traditionally called 'heavy' mitochondria.

■   If the homogenization procedure permits the retention of intact Golgi tubules, these may be approximately 2 μm in length. If the entire stacked Golgi structure is retained then this will sediment with the heavy mitochondria.

Since the velocity of sedimentation of a particle is proportional to d^2, it is principally the size of the particle which determines the rate at which it sediments in a centrifugal field. Velocity of sedimentation (see Equation 2 in Chapter 1) is, however, also determined by the difference in density between that of the particle and that of the liquid ($\rho_p - \rho_l$). The magnitude of this parameter also varies between different subcellular particles; it is largest for nuclei (approximately 0.2 g ml^{-1}) and smallest for Golgi membranes (approximately 0.05 g ml^{-1}). While the difference between these values is significant, the differences in d^2 are greater (*Table 6.2*). Nevertheless, the low density of Golgi membrane tubules is doubtlessly responsible for their anomalously slow sedimentation rate (Section 4), just as the high density of the nuclei contributes to their very rapid sedimentation velocity. The density of subcellular particles is described in more detail in Section 5.

Note that while values for the dimensions of particles can be ascertained reasonably unambiguously in the light and electron microscope, values for their density can only be derived operationally. The density of these particles can only be measured by gradient centrifugation and a true density in a standard homogenate (in 0.25 M sucrose) can only be obtained in a gradient which is isoosmotic (such as iodixanol or Percoll®) not one which is hyperosmotic (such as sucrose).

4. Differential centrifugation of a rat liver homogenate

The technique of differential centrifugation is best illustrated by considering its application to the isolation of crude subcellular fractions from a liver homogenate produced by Potter–Elvehjem homogenization in 0.25 M sucrose, 1 mM EDTA, 10 mM Tris–HCl, pH 7.4. (*Figure 6.4*). Centrifugation at approximately 1000 g for 10 min will pellet the largest particles. Although this pellet is described as the 'nuclear' pellet it will also contain any large sheets of membrane if these are present (Section 4.1). Some of the largest (and densest) mitochondria may also be recovered in this pellet.

The supernatant above the nuclear pellet is decanted and recentrifuged at a higher relative centrifugal field (RCF); commonly this is 3000 g, again for 10 min. This 'heavy' mitochondrial pellet contains predominantly mito-chondria, with rather few contaminating particles. The supernatant is then recentrifuged at 15 000 g for 20 min to pellet the remaining mitochondria, together with the lysosomes and peroxisomes. This pellet, which is com-monly termed the 'light mitochondrial pellet', will also contain most of the tubular Golgi membranes and some of the rough endoplasmic reticulum. The precise magnitude of the RCF and the centrifugation time used to produce the 'light mitochondrial pellet' is rather variable, the RCF may be between 12 000 and 18 000 g and the time from 10–20 min. Centrifugation of the 15 000 g supernatant at 100 000 g for 30–60 min produces the micro-somal pellet which contains all of the remaining membrane vesicles. The

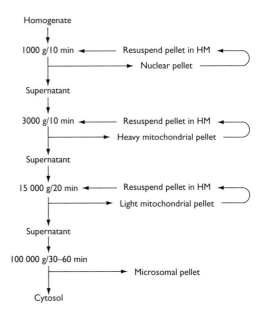

Figure 6.4

Typical differential centrifugation scheme for a rat liver homogenate. The cycle of pellet resus-pension and recentrifugation at the same RCF and time is sometimes termed 'washing the pellet' to remove trapped smaller particles. The two supernatants so produced are combined and passed to the next stage of the differential centrifugation process. Sometimes this cycle is repeated. HM, homogenization medium.

100 000 g supernatant is the cytosolic fraction. As described in Chapter 1 the efficacy of this fractionation process is improved by 'washing the pellets' at each stage to remove smaller particles that pellet anomalously.

4.1 Nuclear pellet

Because their size (and density) and consequently their rate of sedimentation is so very much greater than that of the other organelles, nuclei are normally recovered in high yield and in a relatively pure state in the 1000 g pellet. Contamination by the most rapidly sedimenting mitochondria is, however, significant, but can be virtually eliminated by reducing the RCF to 500 g (although this also reduces the yield of nuclei by approximately one-third). Because of the difference in the rate of sedimentation of these two organelles, the 1000-g pellet is often observed to comprise two overlapping layers, the mitochondria being in the upper layer, which is far less compacted than the lower layer of nuclei. The distinction between these two layers is sufficiently great that the upper layer can be resuspended in medium independently of the lower compact layer if care is taken during the addition and agitation of the medium. This strategy of 'differential resuspension' of an upper less compact layer needs some practice but it may be a useful intermediate purification step.

Technical variation

Disruption of the liver using a loose-fitting Dounce homogenizer in a medium containing 1 mM $MgCl_2$, rather than EDTA, favors the recovery of plasma membrane sheets in the nuclear pellet. One of the earliest published methods for the isolation of plasma membrane, published by Neville (1968), used this approach. If the homogenate is centrifuged in a conical glass tube at 1200 g for 10 min, the pellet is clearly tripartite comprising an upper, very loose, layer of brown mitochondria, a middle creamy layer of plasma membrane sheets and a lower layer of nuclei and cell debris. In the method, the supernatant and the top layer of the pellet were aspirated and discarded and then the middle layer of plasma membranes was resuspended in fresh medium carefully layered onto the residual pellet.

Later this method was refined by placing the total resuspended low-speed pellet on top of a continuous sucrose gradient in order to separate the three components on a rate-zonal basis. The restriction of the volume of sample which can be processed on each gradient (Chapter 1) and the need to produce multiple continuous gradients, led to the use of low-speed zonal rotors for this task (Wisher and Evans, 1975). These rotors are no longer available commercially and the process of isolating the plasma membrane sheets is now largely carried out by density-barrier centrifugation (Hubbard *et al.*, 1983). The initial differential centrifugation is modified in order to eliminate most of the potential contamination from nuclei and mitochondria prior to the density-barrier step (Section 5.8).

4.2 Heavy mitochondrial pellet

The sedimenting properties of the heavy mitochondria are also sufficiently different from those of the particles of the nuclear and light mitochondrial fractions that this fraction is relatively pure, even though it represents only a fraction of the total mitochondria.

Technical variation

If the homogenization is carried out using a Polytron homogenizer, a 5000 *g* pellet produced (without an initial 1000 *g* step) is clearly stratified and the membranes contained in the uppermost layer can be gently resuspended to provide a source of intact, stacked Golgi membranes (Section 5.6).

Preparation of mitochondria for respiratory studies

The most important consideration for respiratory and functional studies is that the method should be as rapid as possible with the minimum number of operations; yields are usually relatively unimportant in the case of a mammalian tissue such as rat liver or beef heart (common sources of mitochondria for these studies). For these purposes, differential centrifugation is commonly used to prepare a heavy mitochondrial fraction, which is relatively little contaminated by other organelles. The presence of free fatty acids in the mitochondria can cause uncoupling so it very important to remove as much lipid as possible during the washing procedure (see *Protocol 6.1*).

■   For more information on the media and isolation procedures from a variety of tissues, see Rice and Lindsay (1997).

4.3   Light mitochondrial pellet

This is so heterogeneous that it can act only as a source of mitochondria, lysosomes, peroxisomes and Golgi membranes for further gradient purification (Section 5).

Practical note

To maximize the recoveries of mitochondria, lysosomes, peroxisomes and Golgi membranes by density-gradient purification, the 3000 *g* step of the differential centrifugation scheme might be omitted.

4.4   Microsomal pellet

Since the size of the majority of the microsomes is so much smaller than that of the particles in the light mitochondrial fraction, the difference in RCF (and time) required to pellet these two types of particle is sufficient to ensure that little or no microsomes are lost at the lower *g*-force and contamination of the 100 000 *g* pellet by residual amounts of lysosomes and peroxisomes *et cetera* which have not pelleted in the 15 000 *g* step is reasonably small. The microsomal pellet, while being an extremely heterogeneous one in terms of the source of the vesicles, is nevertheless reasonably pure (inasmuch as it consists almost entirely of membrane vesicles) and of high yield.

4.5   Behavior of other tissues and cells

The differential centrifugation procedure and the composition of the four pellets as described above are broadly applicable to all tissues and cells. Some of its features, however, are not valid to all systems.

Sheets of rapidly sedimenting plasma membrane, which are derived from the paired contiguous membranes from adjacent hepatocytes and include the bile canalicular domain, are clearly unique to liver. Junctional and desmosomal complexes at the hepatocyte surface stabilize the contiguous domain against fragmentation during homogenization and it is these, and other plasma membrane-associated structures in other tissues, that also promote the production of domain-specific sheets. The luminal brush border (microvillar) membrane of the cells of the intestinal mucosa is also separated from the basolateral domain by junctional complexes, which together with the extensive array of cytoskeletal fibers prevents fragmentation of this domain during homogenization. Cultured cells, on the other hand, never (or very rarely) produce large sheets of plasma membrane since there are few morphological specializations extensive enough to stabilize them.

- ■ The recovery of tubular elements of the Golgi apparatus in the light mitochondrial pellet is also more typical of a tissue such as mammalian liver than of cultured cells whose Golgi membranes normally vesiculate during homogenization.
- ■ 'Heavy' mitochondria are also usually confined to the homogenates of liver, heart and skeletal muscle; homogenates of cultured cells tend to have rather poorly defined mitochondrial fractions in comparison to these tissues.
- ■ Organelles from yeast and other nonphotosynthetic eukaryotes tend to behave in a broadly similar manner to those from animal cells.

4.6 Plant tissues

In a basic text such as this it is not realistic to consider plant tissues in any detail since the methods are very specifically tailored to one particular organelle from a particular species. Thus, for example, the type of medium used and the crude processing of the homogenate for the isolation of chloroplasts from spinach leaves is quite distinctive from that for the isolation of mitochondria from pea seedlings. Because the study of chloroplasts is such an important area of plant research, however, it is worth considering a few of the points that are critical to the success of organelle isolation.

Chloroplasts

The proper selection of the correct species of plant and the choice of tissue are important because of the presence in some plant tissues of high levels of oxalates, phenols and starch which are deleterious the recovery of functioning chloroplasts.

In a crude differential centrifugation scheme, chloroplasts, which are relatively large organelles, will sediment at RCFs similar to those used for nuclei. Consequently, it is common to remove the nuclei not by centrifugation but by (often repeated) filtration of the homogenate (sometimes called a 'brei') through several layers of muslin or combined muslin and cotton wool layers.

Chloroplasts then can be sedimented at 1500–6000 g for 30–60 s. Chloroplast (and other plant organelle) pellets are particularly fragile and the sort of treatments that are routinely used to resuspend mammalian cell organelles (pipeting or liquid shear with a loose-fitting Dounce homogenizer) are never used, a soft-haired paint brush being the instrument of choice.

Other plant organelles such as mitochondria and peroxisomes (microbodies) and those from fungi and yeast are normally pelleted at similar RCFs to those from animal cells, although the media that are used are very different and usually contain a slightly higher concentration (0.3 M) of an osmotic balancer than is routinely used for mammalian liver, which may be sucrose but more commonly is either mannitol or sorbitol.

5.   Purification of organelles in gradients

5.1   Density of organelles in different media

Generally speaking, neither yields nor purities are sufficiently high for differential centrifugation to be used as the sole means of fractionation, and gradient centrifugation is a necessary procedure.

In sucrose

A casual search through the current literature will reveal that sucrose has more or less retained its place as one of the principal gradient media for subcellular organelles. This is largely due to the huge number of published methods which have accumulated over several decades. It is, however, far from ideal for separating the major organelles. Principally because of the high osmolality of sucrose gradients, osmotically active organelles (nuclei, mitochondria and lysosomes) lose water during their passage through such gradients and consequently steadily increase in density until they approach a limiting value. The density of peroxisomes also increases as they sediment through the gradient but not because of the rising osmolarity. Peroxisomes are permeable to sucrose and thus their density is a composite of the density of the molecules of the organelles and the sucrose which enters them (*Table 6.3*).

The difficulty in resolving lysosomes in sucrose led workers to use a density-perturbation technique to lower the density of these organelles artificially. The method involves injecting an experimental animal with Triton WR1339 (Leighton *et al.*, 1968) – a nonionic detergent that is taken up into lysosomes and consequently makes them less dense. This dubious practice can now be avoided by use of one of the media of lower osmolality.

Nuclei, because of their DNA content, have a distinctively high density, while Golgi membranes tend to have a uniquely low density (they have the highest lipid:protein ratio of any membrane beside myelin), consequently they can be well separated from other membranes, even in sucrose gradients (Sections 5.2 and 5.6). Although plasma membrane sheets have a density

Table 6.3. Density (g ml^{-1}) of organelles in different gradient media

Organelle	Sucrose	Nycodenz®	Iodixanol	Percoll®
Nuclei	>1.30	1.24–1.26	1.22–1.24	na
Mitochondria	1.17–1.21	1.16–1.19	1.14–1.16	1.08–1.10
Lysosomes	1.19–1.21	1.12–1.14	1.11–1.14	1.10–1.11
Peroxisomes	1.18–1.23	1.18–1.21	1.17–1.21	1.07–1.08
Golgi membranes	1.05–1.12	1.06–1.12	1.03–1.08	1.03–1.10
Plasma membrane sheets	1.14–1.19	1.11–1.15	na	na

na, not available.

range which overlaps that of mitochondria, *et cetera*, because they can be recovered at a lower RCF during differential centrifugation, this is not a major problem.

In iodinated density-gradient media and Percoll®

In media such as iodixanol and Percoll®, whose gradients can be made iso-osmotic over the entire useful density range (Chapter 3), osmotically sensitive organelles retain their enclosed water space and are consequently much less dense than in sucrose and the density range of each organelle type generally allows for better resolution than with sucrose (*Table 6.3*). In Nycodenz®, the mitochondria and the nuclei band at densities that are slightly hyperosmotic, and hence are slightly higher than in iodixanol. In comparing the efficacy of the two iodinated density-gradient media, this may actually be beneficial to the separation of lysosomes and mitochondria, while the slightly lower density of mitochondria in iodixanol is beneficial to the separation of peroxisomes and mitochondria. In Percoll®, the densities of all organelles are lower than in either Nycodenz® or iodixanol and the sequence of organelles and density is reversed. This is clearly a function of the different nature of these media (colloid vs. true solute); the actual reason, however, is not at all clear, although the lower density of peroxisomes in Percoll® is doubtless related to the fact that the internal compartment of these organelles is freely available to small molecules but not to colloidal silica.

■   Since peroxisomes do not have an osmotically active compartment, their density in sucrose, Nycodenz® and iodixanol is rather similar.

Practical notes

Percoll® is commonly (but not exclusively) used as a self-generated gradient for organelle separations while both Nycodenz® and iodixanol tend to be used predominantly as preformed continuous or discontinuous gradients. Iodixanol can be used in a self-generated gradient but the RCFs required ($>180\,000\ g$) are higher than those needed for Percoll® and higher than the routine RCFs used for gradient centrifugation of organelles. Nevertheless, because of the convenience of using a self-generated gradient and the high resolving power of iodixanol for peroxisomes, a protocol for these organelles using such a gradient is included for completeness. See Chapter 3 for more information about these gradient media.

In the following sections, the methods of purifying nuclei and the major organelles of the light mitochondrial fraction (Section 4.3) will be considered. Sometimes it is not necessary to prepare specific organelles from the light mitochondrial fraction (or heavy + light mitochondrial fraction) but to devise an 'analytical' gradient in which the requirement is that each organelle should have a distinctive banding pattern against which the distribution of some functional or compositional parameter may be compared. It is not, however, necessary that the gradient produces high-purity fractions of each organelle – indeed such a result is probably beyond the capability of any single gradient (Section 5.7).

5.2   Nuclei

Because of their DNA content, nuclei have a distinctive high density, which makes it relatively easily to purify them from other organelles using simple discontinuous density gradients or density barriers. It is customary, but no essential, to isolate a crude nuclear fraction first (Section 4.1) in buffered 0.25 M sucrose containing 25 mM KCl and 5 mM $MgCl_2$ in order to maintain the nuclei in a condensed state. Where this is not possible, for example certain cultured cells will only homogenize in an EDTA containing medium the density of the nuclei may be found to be reduced.

■   If EDTA is a prerequisite for efficient homogenization of a cultured cell line, then KCl and $MgCl_2$ should be added to the suspending medium as soon as possible after homogenization.

Sucrose density-barrier centrifugation

The 'traditional manner' in which nuclei are purified is to resuspend the nuclear pellet from an homogenate in 60% (w/w) sucrose (Blobel and Potter, 1966). Because of the residual liquid in the pellet, the density of the sucrose solution is reduced so that it can be layered over a density barrier of 60% sucrose. After centrifugation at 100 000 g for 2 h, only the nuclei are sufficiently dense (>1.32 g ml^{-1}) to sediment through the 60% ($\rho = 1.2865$ g ml^{-1}) sucrose barrier (*Protocol 6.2*). Because of the osmolal ity of the medium, however, the nuclei condense considerably in size and this is the reason for their very high density in sucrose. Indeed, the actual density of nuclei in sucrose is not accurately known and only a lower limit value (>1.32 g ml^{-1}) is normally quoted. The high viscosity of the sucrose medium also means that their rate of sedimentation is slow and conse quently centrifugation times are long.

This separation illustrates two useful practices that minimize aggregation of particles at an interface.

■   By suspending the crude nuclear pellet in a medium, which has a density of 1.22–1.24 g ml^{-1}, any contaminating organelles of a lower density will tend to float to the surface and only the nuclei will sediment.

■   Large density differences between adjacent layers should be avoided to prevent a sudden reduction in particle sedimentation rate and conse quent build-up and aggregation of particles at the interface.

Discontinuous iodixanol gradient

The density of nuclei in an isoosmotic medium such as iodixanol is signifi cantly lower (1.20–1.22 g ml^{-1}) than that in sucrose, consequently the con centrations of iodixanol required are much lower and much less viscous so that sedimentation takes place more rapidly. Moreover, it is possible to arrange that the nuclei band above a density barrier rather than form a pellet as is the case with sucrose (Graham *et al.*, 1994). If a whole homogenate is adjusted to a density of approximately 1.14 g ml^{-1} and layered over two density barriers ($\rho = 1.175$ and 1.20 g ml^{-1}) and if the RCF is kept suffi ciently low (10 000 g for 20 min), then although the density range of per oxisomes overlaps that of nuclei in iodixanol, because of their much smaller size they sediment much more slowly, so that at this low RCF all of the other organelles in the homogenate remain in the topmost layer and only the nuclei have both a sufficiently high density and sedimentation rate to reach the interface between the two barriers (*Figure 6.5* and *Protocol 6.3*).

■   For more information on the isolation of nuclei, nuclear membranes and nuclear subfractions, see Rickwood *et al.* (1997).

5.3   Mitochondria

Because of the huge literature on sucrose gradients, it is worth noting that one of the most successful methods (Diczfalusy and Alexson, 1988) uses a continuous 34–54% (w/v) sucrose, containing 1 mM EDTA, 10 mM Hepes–NaOH, pH 7.4; the crude fraction is layered on top and centrifuged at 150 000 g for 45 min. The mitochondria band in the middle of the gradient. Discontinuous sucrose gradients of 30, 40 and 55% (w/v) sucrose (Beauvoit *et al.*, 1989) are an alternative (mitochondria band at the 40/55% interface) and are often used for yeast. However, modern isoosmotic media are becoming increasingly adopted as a gentle means of preparing mitochondria.

Percoll®

Because of the relatively low RCFs that are needed for the formation of Percoll® gradients, a popular approach is to layer a crude mitochondrial fraction onto a 30% (v/v) solution of Percoll® (containing 225 mM mannitol). Gradient formation is normally carried out in a fixed-angle rotor at 95 000 g (*Protocol 6.4*). The mitochondria band at approximately 1.09 g ml^{-1} (Hovius *et al.*, 1990).

It is important that the fraction used contains as little endoplasmic reticulum (ER) as possible, since in Percoll® gradients the density of mitochondria and ER tend to overlap quite significantly (Patel *et al.*, 1991), thus the post-nuclear supernatant should be centrifuged at 10 000 g rather than higher RCFs.

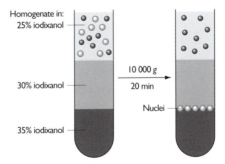

Figure 6.5

Purification of nuclei from an homogenate in a discontinuous iodixanol gradient. Under the centrifugation conditions only the nuclei are dense enough and sufficiently rapidly sedimenting at 10 000 g to reach the lower interface. The other organelles remain in the load zone.

An alternative approach, which permits the use of ER-containing fractions, is to use a pre-formed four-step discontinuous gradient of Percoll (Reinhart *et al.*, 1982). A total homogenate can be used and the centrifugation at 37 000 *g* is carried out in a swinging-bucket rotor for only 30 s. The separation relies on the use of sedimentation rate to prevent the smaller particles from reaching their banding density. The procedure is, however, very restrictive since only 2 ml of homogenate can be processed on a single 11-ml gradient.

Iodixanol

An effective way of using a pre-formed gradient is to use a short sedimentation path-length vertical rotor (Chapter 2) so as to minimize both the centrifugation time and the RCF. This also reduces the hydrostatic pressure experienced by the organelles. A light mitochondrial fraction is layered over a 13–45% (w/v) iodixanol gradient and centrifuged at 32 000 *g* for 75 min in a Beckman VTi50 rotor (Solaas *et al.*, 2000).

■   Note that a small volume of dense medium underlies the gradient to prevent dense particles reaching the wall of the tube.

5.4 Peroxisomes

Although in Percoll® peroxisomes are the least dense of the major organelles (Section 5.1) and band away from mitochondria and lysosomes, the ER which always contaminates the light mitochondrial fraction has the same buoyant density and cannot therefore be resolved from peroxisomes. This is not the case with iodixanol in which peroxisomes are the densest organelle, and any ER bands at much lower densities. Iodixanol is certainly the medium of choice for peroxisomes and Van Veldhoven *et al.* (1996) devised a pre-formed continuous gradient of iodixanol (*Protocol 6.5*). Because of the high linear separation of the peroxisomes from the other organelles (*Figure 6.6*), it is possible to carry out this separation in a fixed-angle rotor rather than a swinging-bucket rotor, thus increasing the material capacity of the system. The gradient solutions are constructed such that the gradient of iodixanol also contains a negative gradient of sucrose and in this manner the density gradient is maintained isoosmotic over the entire density range (see Chapter 3).

Practical notes

Low concentrations of ethanol in all media are beneficial to the recovery of functionally intact peroxisomes: a commonly used homogenization medium is 0.25 M sucrose, 1 mM EDTA, 0.1% (v/v) ethanol, 5 mM Mops–NaOH pH 7.2.

■   Iodixanol can also be effectively used in a self-generated mode for isolation of peroxisomes (See Notes to Protocol 6.5).

5.5 Lysosomes

Percoll ®

In Percoll®, lysosomes are the densest of the major organelles and consequently relatively easy to isolate. Although the lysosomes are obtained in a high purity, yields tend to be relatively low (less than 60%). The less-dense

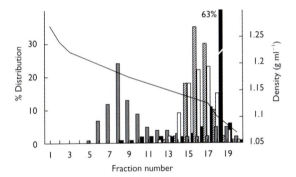

Figure 6.6

Separation of peroxisomes in a pre-formed continuous iodixanol gradient: percentage distribution of enzyme markers. The method is described in Protocol 6.5; *density (——), glucose-6–phosphatase (■), catalase (■), acid phosphatase (□), glutamate dehydrogenase (▨); markers for endoplasmic reticulum, peroxisomes, lysosomes and mitochondria respectively. Reproduced from Van Veldhoven et al. (1996)* Anal. Biochem. **237**; *17–23, with kind permission of the authors and Academic Press.*

lysosomes in particular which band towards the middle of the gradient are contaminated by the other organelles and consequently not recoverable (*Figure 6.7*). As with the isolation of peroxisomes, the light mitochondrial fraction is layered on top of a uniform concentration of Percoll® and centrifuged in a fixed-angle rotor to generate a gradient (Symons and Jonas, 1987). The method is given in *Protocol 6.6*.

Nycodenz®

As an alternative to the self-generated Percoll® gradient, a light mitochondrial fraction can be adjusted to a high density by mixing with a stock Nycodenz® solution and layering under a discontinuous gradient of Nycodenz® (Wattiaux and Wattiaux-De Coninck, 1983; Olsson *et al.*, 1989).

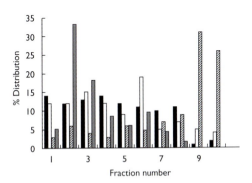

Figure 6.7

Separation of lysosomes in a self-generated gradient of Percoll®: percentage distribution of enzyme markers. The method is described in Protocol 6.6; *catalase (■), glucose-6–phosphatase (■), cytochrome oxidase (□), β-hexosaminidase (▨); markers for peroxisomes, endoplasmic reticulum, mitochonria and lysosomes respectively (gradient unloaded dense end first). Data adapted from Symons and Jonas (1987)* Anal. Biochem. **164**; *382–390.*

In this medium, the lysosomes will float to the top of the gradient during centrifugation and the separation from mitochondria is probably better than that obtained with iodixanol (*Protocol 6.7*).

5.6   Golgi membranes

When using a tissue such as liver, in which the Golgi membranes form very well-defined stacks of tubular membranes, homogenization in the presence of dextran promotes the retention of these stacks. It is also important to use a Polytron™ type of homogenizer, which disrupts the tissue by mechanical shear forces rather then a liquid shear device. These intact Golgi stacks from mammalian liver can be sedimented at 5000 *g* and subsequently purified by banding at a 1.2-M sucrose barrier (Morré *et al.*, 1972). Subsequently the Golgi can be 'unstacked' by hydrolyzing the dextran with a mixture of amylases. The method (*Protocol 6.8*) is less successful with cultured cells which exhibit a less extensive and organized Golgi system (see Chapter 7).

In the absence of dextran the Golgi tubules in the light mitochondrial fraction can be isolated by flotation through a discontinuous sucrose gradient (Fleischer and Fleischer, 1970). The light mitochondrial fraction is adjusted to 1.55 M sucrose and 4–5 ml overlaid with the following sucrose solutions: 2.5 ml of 1.33 M, 2 ml of 1.2 M and 1.1 M, and 1 ml of 0.77 M and 0.25 M sucrose. After centrifugation at 160 000 g_{av} for 1 h, the Golgi bands at the top two interfaces.

Graham and Winterbourne (1988) subsequently adapted this system to an iodinated density gradient medium. The Golgi membranes are allowed to float from a 30% Nycodenz® layer through a discontinuous gradient of 25, 20, 15 and 10% (w/v) Nycodenz® during centrifugation at 250 000g for 4 h. The 10 and 15% layers resolve functionally distinct low-density and high-density subpopulations of Golgi membranes.

5.7   An analytical system for the light mitochondrial fraction

Because of the potentially high resolving power of an isoosmotic gradient, it is possible to obtain good separations of all the major organelles of the light mitochondrial fraction in a continuous gradient. This can be accomplished by flotation through a performed linear gradient of iodixanol or Nycodenz® (Graham *et al.*, 1994). If the light mitochondria is layered beneath a 10–30% (w/v) iodixanol gradient then centrifuged at 70 000 *g* for 1.5–2 h, each major organelle bands distinctively in the gradient without unacceptable overlap (*Figure 6.8*). *Protocol 6.9* gives a self-generated gradient as an interesting alternative. Any analytical study to investigate the localization of a particular component or function to one or more membrane particles either temporally or under different conditions may require the production of several identical gradients. Not only are self-generated gradients easier to prepare, they are also highly reproducible. The 17.5% iodixanol gradient described in *Protocol 6.9* has also been used as a method for purifying lysosomes (Gille and Nohl, 2000).

5.8   Plasma membrane sheets

When rat liver is homogenized under isoosmotic conditions in an Mg^{2-}-containing medium using very gentle Dounce homogenization, the contiguous plasma membranes from adjacent parenchymal cells are released as

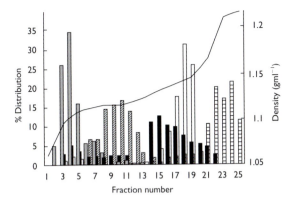

Figure 6.8

Fractionation (analytical) of a light mitochondrial fraction in a pre-formed iodixanol gradient: percentage distribution of enzyme markers. Density (——), catalase (⊟),succinate dehydrogenase (▢), β-galactosidase (■), NADPH-cytochrome c-reductase (▨), UDP-galactose galactosyltransferase (▩); markers for peroxisomes, mitochondria, lysosomes, endoplasmic reticulum and Golgi respectively.

large paired sheets which can be isolated by low-speed centrifugation and purified by flotation through a simple density barrier (*Protocol 6.10*).

References

Balch, W.E., Dunphy, W.G., Braell, W.A. and Rothman, J.E. (1984) Reconstitution of the transport of protein between successive compartments of the Golgi measured by the coupled incorporation of N-acetylglucosamine. *Cell* **39**: 405–416.

Beauvoit, B. Rigoulet, M. Guerin, B. and Canioni, P. (1989) Polyphosphates, a source of high energy phosphate in yeast mitochondria: a ^{31}P NMR study. *FEBS Lett.* **252**: 17–21.

Blobel, G. and Potter, V.R. (1966) Nuclei from rat liver: an isolation method that combines purity with high yield. *Science* **154**: 1662–1665.

Diczfalusy, U. and Alexson, S.E.H. (1988) Peroxisomal chain shortening of prostaglandin F_2. *J. Lipid Res.* **29**: 1629–1636.

Fleischer, B. and Fleischer, S. (1970) Preparation and characterization of Golgi membranes from rat liver. *Biochim. Biophys. Acta* **219**: 301–319.

Gille, L. and Nohl, H. (2000) The existence of a lysosomal redox cain and the role of ubiqinone. *Arch. Biochem. Biophys.* **375**: 347–354.

Goldberg, D.E. and Korafeld, S. (1983) Evidence for extensive subcellular organization of asparagine-linked oligosaccharide processing and lysososomal enzyme phosphorylation. *J. Biol. Chem.* **258**: 3159–3165.

Graham, J.M. (1997) Homogenization of tissues and cells. In: *Subcellular Fractionation – A Practical Approach* (eds. J.M. Graham and D. Rickwood). IRL Press at Oxford University Press, Oxford, pp. 1–29.

Graham, J.M. and Winterbourne, D.J. (1988) Subcellular localization of the sulphation reaction of heparan sulphate synthesis and transport of the proteoglycan to the cell surface of rat liver. *Biochem. J.* **252**: 437–445.

Graham, J., Ford, T. and Rickwood, D. (1994) The preparation of subcellular organelles from mouse liver in self-generated gradients of iodixanol. *Anal. Biochem.* **220**: 367–373.

Hovius, R., Lambrechts, H., Nicolay, K. and de Kruijff, B. (1990) Improved methods to isolate and subfractionate rat liver mitochondria. Lipid composition of the inner and outer membrane. *Biochim. Biophys. Acta* **102**: 217–226.

Hubbard, A.L., Wall, D.A. and Ma, A. (1983) Isolation of rat hepatocyte plasma membranes. I Presence of three major domains. *J. Cell Biol.* **96**: 217–229.

Leighton, F., Poole, B., Beaufay, H., Baudhuin, P., Coffey, J.W., Fowler, S. and de Duve, C. (1968) The large scale separation of peroxisomes, mitochondria and lysosomes from the livers of rats injected with Triton WR 1339. *J. Cell Biol.* **37**: 482–513.

Moore, A.L., Fricaud, A-C., Walters, A.J. and Whitehouse, D.G. (1993) Isolation of purification of functionally intact mitochondria from plant cells. In: *Methods in Molecular Biology*, Vol. 19 (eds J.M. Graham and J.A. Higgins). Humana Press, Totowa, NJ, pp. 133–139.

Morré, D. J., Cheetham, R. D. and Nyquist, S. E. (1972) A simplified procedure for isolation of Golgi apparatus from rat liver. *Prep. Biochem.* **2**: 61–66.

Neville, D.M. (1968) Isolation of an organ-specific protein antigen from the cell surface membrane of rat liver. *Biochim. Biophys. Acta* **154**: 540–552.

Olsson, G.M., Svensson, I., Zdoisek, J.M. and Brunk, U.T. (1989) Lysosomal enzyme leakage during the hypoxanthine/xanthine oxidase reaction. *Virchows Archiv. B Cell Pathol.* **56**: 385–391.

Patel, B., Costi, A., Hardy, L. and Mowbray, J. (1991) The characterization of a new enzyme from rat liver mitochondria, oligophosphoglyceroyl-ATP 3′-phosphodiesterase. *Biochem. J.* **274**: 275–279.

Preller, A. and Wilson, J.E. (1992) Localization of the type III isozyme of hexokinase at the nuclear periphery. *Arch. Biochem. Biophys.* **294**: 482–492.

Reinhart, P.H., Taylor, W.M. and Bygrave, F.L. (1982) A procedure for the rapid preparation of mitochondria from rat liver. *Biochem. J.* **204**: 731–735.

Rice, J.E. and Lindsay, J.G. (1997) Subcellular fractionation of mitochondria. In: *Subcellular Fractionation – A Practical Approach* (eds J.M. Graham and D. Rickwood). IRL Press at Oxford University Press, Oxford, pp. 107–142.

Rickwood, D., Messent, A. and Patel, D. (1997) Isolation and characterization of nuclei and nuclear subfractions. In: *Subcellular Fractionation – A Practical Approach* (eds J.M. Graham and D. Rickwood). IRL Press at Oxford University Press, Oxford, pp. 71–105.

Solaas, K., Ulvestad, A., Söreide, O. and Kase, B.F. (2000) Subcellular organization of bile acid amidation in human liver: a key issue in regulating the biosythesis of bile salts. *J. Lipid Res.* **41**: 1154–1162.

Symons, L.J. and Jonas, A.J. (1987) Isolation of highly purified rat liver lysosomal membranes using two Percoll gradients. *Anal. Biochem.* **164**: 382–390.

Van Veldhoven, P.P., Baumgart, E. and Mannaerts, G.P. (1996) Iodixanol (OptiPrep™), an improved density gradient medium for the iso-osmotic isolation of rat liver peroxisomes. *Anal. Biochem.* **237**: 17–23.

Wattiaux, R. and Wattiaux-De Coninck S. (1983) Separation of cell organelles. In: *Iodinated Density Gradient Media – A Practical Approach* (ed. D. Rickwood). IRL Press at Oxford University Press, Oxford, pp. 119–137.

Whitehouse, D.G. and Moore, A.L. (1993) Isolation of purification of functionally intact chloroplasts from leaf tissue and leaf tissue protoplasts. In: *Methods in Molecular Biology* Vol. 19 (eds J.M. Graham and J.A. Higgins). Humana Press, Totowa, NJ, pp. 123–131.

Wisher, M. H. and Evans, W.H. (1975) Functional polarity of the rat hepatocyte surface membrane. *Biochem. J.* **146**: 375–388.

Protocol 6.1

Isolation of rat liver mitochondria by differential centrifugation

Equipment

Overhead electric motor, thyristor-controlled, mounted either to a wall, via a G-clamp to the bench or in a floor-standing cradle

Potter–Elvehjem homogenizer (20–30 ml: clearance approximately 0.09 mm)

Dounce homogenizer (loose-fitting Wheaton type B pestle, approximately 30 ml)

High-speed centrifuge with fixed-angle rotor for 40–50 ml clear polycarbonate tubes

Low-speed refrigerated centrifuge with swinging-bucket rotor for 50 ml tubes.

Reagents

Homogenization medium (HM): 0.2 M mannitol, 0.05 M sucrose, 10 mM KCl, 1 mM EDTA, 10 mM Hepes–NaOH, pH 7.4.

Protocol

Keep all equipment and all solutions in ice before use and carry out all operations at 0–4°C. This protocol is designed for a liver from one adult male rat.

1. Kill the experimental animal (starved overnight) by cervical dislocation or decapitation. This must be supervised or carried out by an experienced animal technician.

2. Remove the liver to a beaker containing about 30 ml of HM.

3. Decant the medium and with the beaker in ice, finely mince the liver using scissors.

4. Suspend the mince in 40 ml of HM and transfer about half the suspension to the glass vessel of the Potter–Elvehjem homogenizer.

5. Homogenize the liver with 7–8 strokes of the pestle (at 500–700 r.p.m.).

6. Rinse the homogenizer with medium to remove any connective tissue that may be adhering and repeat the procedure with the other half of the mince.

7. Centrifuge the homogenate at 1000 g_{av} for 10 min in the low speed centrifuge.

8. Distribute the supernatant between two 40–50 ml polycarbonate tubes.

9. Centrifuge at 3000g_{av} for 10 min (high-speed centrifuge).

10. Aspirate the supernatant from each tube removing as much of the floating lipid layer as possible and also the loose-packed pinkish layer that overlies the brown mitochondria.

11. Wipe away any remaining lipid adhering to the wall of the tube.

12. Add a small amount of HM to each pellet and crudely resuspend the pellet with a glass rod.

13. Resuspend the pellet fully using three or four gentle strokes of the pestle of the Dounce homogenizer and dilute to the original volume.

14. Transfer to new centrifuge tubes and repeat the centrifugation and pellet washing twice more.

15. Finally resuspend the purified mitochondria in a suitable buffer or HM as required.

Protocol 6.2

Isolation of rat liver nuclei in a sucrose gradient (Blobel and Potter, 1996)

Equipment

Overhead electric motor, thyristor-controlled, mounted either to a wall, via a G-clamp to the bench or in a floor-standing cradle

Potter–Elvehjem homogenizer (20–30 ml: clearance approximately 0.09 mm)

Dounce homogenizer (loose-fitting Wheaton type B pestle, approximately 30 ml)

Low-speed centrifuge with fixed-angle rotor for 40–50 ml tubes

Ultracentrifuge with swinging-bucket rotor for approximately 14 ml tubes (e.g. Beckman SW41)

Refractometer

Nylon gauze or cheesecloth.

Reagents

Homogenization medium (HM): 0.25 M sucrose, 25 mM KCl, 5 mM $MgCl_2$, 10 mM Hepes–NaOH, pH 7.4 (SKM)

Density medium: 2.3 M sucrose 25 mM KCl, 5 mM $MgCl_2$, 10 mM Hepes–NaOH, pH 7.4.

Protocol

Keep all equipment and all solutions in ice before use and carry out all operations at 0–4°C. This protocol is designed for a liver from one adult male rat.

1. Prepare an homogenate as described in steps 1–6 of *Protocol 6.1* using SKM as homogenization medium.

2. Filter the homogenate through a single layer of nylon gauze or three layers of cheesecloth to remove any connective tissue. Assist filtration by stirring with a glass rod.

3. Dilute the homogenate with at least an equal volume of SKM.

4. Centrifuge at 1000 g for 10 min.

5. Decant the supernatant; add 2 volumes of the 2.3 M sucrose solution and mix very thoroughly using a loose-fitting Dounce homogenizer.

6. Check that the refractive index of the suspension is 1.4117 ($\pm$0.0004) and adjust if required.

7. Transfer 9 ml of suspension to a 14 ml centrifuge tube; underlayer with 2.3 M sucrose to fill the tube and centrifuge at 130 000 g for 30 min at 4°C in the swinging-bucket rotor.

8. Decant all the liquid from above the pellet and resuspend the latter in SKM.

Protocol 6.3

Isolation of rat liver nuclei in an iodixanol gradient

Equipment

Overhead electric motor, thyristor-controlled, mounted either to a wall, via a G-clamp to the bench or in a floor-standing cradle

Potter-Elvehjem homogenizer (20–30 ml: clearance approximately 0.09 mm)

High-speed centrifuge with swinging-bucket rotor for 40–50 ml tubes

Nylon gauze or cheesecloth.

Reagents

Homogenization medium (HM): SKM (see *Protocol 6.2*)

OptiPrep™

Diluent: 150 mM KCl, 30 mM MgCl₂, 60 mM Hepes–NaOH, pH 7.4

Working solution of 50% (w/v) iodixanol: mix 5 volumes of OptiPrep™ with I volume of diluent.

Protocol

Keep all equipment and all solutions in ice before use and carry out all operations at 0–4°C. This protocol is designed for a liver from one adult male rat.

1. Prepare a filtered homogenate as described in steps 1–3 of *Protocol 6.2* using SKM as homogenization medium.

2. Mix the homogenate with an equal volume of 50% iodixanol working solution.

3. Prepare iodixanol solutions of 30 and 35% (w/v) by dilution of the 50% iodixanol solution with SKM.

4. In a centrifuge tube layer equal volumes (e.g. 15 ml each) of the 35 and 30% iodixanol solutions and overlayer with the approximately 20 ml of the homogenate/25% iodixanol.

5. Centrifuge at 10 000 g_{av} for 20 min at 4°C in the swinging- bucket rotor.

6. Harvest the nuclei from above the 35% iodixanol; dilute with 2 volumes of SKM and centrifuge at 2000 g_{av} for 10 min before resuspending in a suitable medium.

Protocol 6.4

Isolation of rat liver mitochondria in a Percoll® gradient (Hovius *et al.*, 1990)

Equipment

Overhead electric motor, thyristor-controlled, mounted either to a wall, via a G-clamp to the bench or in a floor-standing cradle

Potter–Elvehjem homogenizer (20–30 ml: clearance approximately 0.09 mm)

High-speed centrifuge with fixed-angle rotor for 40–50 ml polycarbonate tubes

Ultracentrifuge and fixed-angle rotor with thick-walled polycarbonate tubes (at least 25 ml, e.g. Beckman 60Ti or equivalent)

Dounce homogenizer (loose-fitting Wheaton type B pestle, approximately 30 ml)

Dounce homogenizer (loose-fitting Wheaton type B pestle, approximately 5 ml).

Reagents

Homogenization medium (HM): 0.25 M mannitol, 0.5 mM EGTA, 0.1% (w/v) bovine serum albumin (BSA), 5 mM Hepes–NaOH, pH 7.4

Percoll®

Diluent: 450 mM mannitol, 2 mM EGTA, 0.2% (w/v) BSA, 50 mM Hepes–NaOH, pH 7.4

Percoll® stock (30%, v/v): dilute 3 volumes of Percoll with 2 volumes of water and 5 volumes of diluent.

Protocol

Keep all equipment and all solutions in ice before use and carry out all operations at 0–4°C. This protocol is designed for a liver from one adult male rat.

1. Produce a post-nuclear (1000 g) supernatant from a rat liver homogenate in the above HM using steps 1–7 of *Protocol 6.1*.

2. Centrifuge the supernatant at 10 000 g for 15 min.

3. Discard the supernatant and resuspend the pellet in HM (approximately 20 ml), using a glass rod, followed by three or four gentle strokes of the pestle of the Dounce homogenizer.

4. Recentrifuge at 15 000 g for 15 min and discard the supernatant.

5. Resuspend the pellet in 5 ml of HM as in step 3.

6. Place 20 ml of the Percoll® stock in each of four tubes for the ultracentrifuge rotor and layer the resuspended pellet on top.

7. Centrifuge at 95 000 g for 30 min.

8. Collect the lower part of the dense brown/yellow band.

9. Dilute the mitochondrial suspension with at least 2 volumes of HM and pellet the organelles at 6300 g for 10 min in the high-speed centrifuge.

10. Wash the mitochondrial pellet at least twice more with HM before resuspending in an appropriate medium.

Protocol 6.5

Isolation of rat liver peroxisomes in a pre-formed iodixanol gradient (Van Velhoven *et al.*, 1996)

Equipment

Overhead electric motor, thyristor-controlled, mounted either to a wall, via a G-clamp to the bench or in a floor-standing cradle

Potter–Elvehjem homogenizer (20–30 ml: clearance approximately 0.09 mm)

High-speed centrifuge with fixed-angle rotor for 40–50 ml polycarbonate tubes

Ultracentrifuge and fixed-angle rotor with thick-walled polycarbonate tubes (at least 25 ml, e.g. Beckman 60Ti or equivalent)

Gradient maker (two-chamber or Gradient Master™)

Gradient unloader for dense end first collection (see Chapter 4)

Dounce homogenizer (loose-fitting Wheaton type B pestle, approximately 30 ml)

Dounce homogenizer (loose-fitting Wheaton type B pestle, approximately 5 ml).

Reagents

Peroxisome homogenization medium (PHM): 0.25 M sucrose, 1 mM EDTA, 0.1% (v/v) ethanol, 5 mM Mops–NaOH pH 7.2

OptiPrep™

Diluent: 6 mM EDTA, 0.6% ethanol, 30 mM Mops–NaOH, pH 7.2

Gradient solutions of 50, 40 and 20% (w/v) iodixanol: prepare from OptiPrep™/diluent/1 M sucrose/water at the following volume ratios: (1) 5:0.6:0.4:0; (2) 4:0.6:0.7:0.7 and (3) 2:0.6:1.1:2.3.

Protocol

Keep all equipment and all solutions in ice before use and carry out all operations at 0–4°C. This protocol is designed for a liver from one adult male rat.

1. Prepare a 3000 *g* supernatant from a liver homogenate in PHM according to steps 1–9 of *Protocol 6.1*.

2. Centrifuge the supernatant in the high-speed centrifuge at 15 000 *g* for 15 min.

3. Discard the supernatant and resuspend the pellet in PHM (approximately 20 ml) using a glass rod and then three or four gentle strokes of the pestle of the Dounce homogenizer.

4. Recentrifuge at 15 000 g for 15 min and discard the supernatant.

5. Suspend the pellet in PHM as in step 3, adjusting to a volume of 0.5 ml g^{-1} of tissue.

6. Prepare two linear gradients from 9 ml each of gradient solutions 2 and 3 in the thick-walled polycarbonate tubes.

7. Underlayer each gradient with 2 ml of gradient solution 1.

8. Layer 3 ml of the light mitochondrial suspension over each gradient and centrifuge at 105 000 g for 1 h.

9. Allow the rotor to decelerate from 1000 r.p.m. without the brake and collect the gradient in 1 ml fractions dense end first.

10. The peak peroxisome fraction is 7–8 ml from the bottom of the gradient.

Note

In the alternative self-generated gradient, the light mitochondrial fraction in step 5 is simply mixed with an equal volume of the 50% iodixanol, transferred to a tube for a vertical, near vertical or low-angle fix-angle rotor and centrifuged at 180 000 g for 2–3 h (the actual time will depend on the rotor). The peroxisomes band in the bottom third of the gradient. For more information see Graham et al., 1994.

Protocol 6.6

Isolation of rat liver lysosomes in a Percoll® gradient (Symons and Jones, 1987)

Equipment

Overhead electric motor, thyristor-controlled, mounted either to a wall, via a G-clamp to the bench or in a floor-standing cradle

Potter–Elvehjem homogenizer (20–30 ml: clearance approximately 0.09 mm)

High-speed centrifuge with fixed-angle rotors for 40–50 ml and 12–15 ml tubes

Dounce homogenizer (loose-fitting Wheaton type B pestle, approximately 30 ml).

Reagents

Lysosome homogenization medium (LHM): 0.25 M sucrose, 1 mM EDTA, 20 mM Hepes–NaOH, pH 7.4

Percoll®

Diluent: 2.5 M sucrose, 10 mM EDTA, 200 mM Hepes–NaOH, pH 7.4 (SEH)

Percoll® stock: (9 volumes of Percoll® + 1 volume of diluent).

Protocol

Keep all equipment and all solutions in ice before use and carry out all operations at 0–4°C. This protocol is designed for a liver from one adult male rat.

1. Prepare a washed light mitochondrial fraction according to steps 1–4 of *Protocol 6.5* using LHM.

2. Suspend the light mitochondrial pellet in 10 ml of LHM.

3. Mix the Percoll® stock with this light mitochondrial suspension (55:45, v/v).

4. Centrifuge at 35 000 g for 90 min (10 ml in each centrifuge tube).

5. Allow the rotor to decelerate from 1000 r.p.m. without the brake and collect the lysosomes which band in the bottom 1–2 ml of the gradient.

6. Dilute the suspension with 5 volumes of SEH and centrifuge at 20 000 g for 10 min to harvest the lysosomes which band just above the gelatinous pellet of Percoll® particles.

Protocol 6.7

Isolation of rat liver lysosomes in a Nycodenz® gradient (Olsson *et al.*, 1989)

Equipment

Overhead electric motor, thyristor-controlled, mounted either to a wall, via a G-clamp to the bench or in a floor-standing cradle

Potter–Elvehjem homogenizer (20–30 ml: clearance approximately 0.09 mm)

High-speed centrifuge with fixed-angle rotors for 40–50 ml tubes

Ultracentrifuge with swinging-bucket rotor for approximately 38 ml tubes (e.g. Beckman SW28)

Dounce homogenizer (loose-fitting Wheaton type B pestle, approximately 30 ml)

Dounce homogenizer (loose-fitting Wheaton type B pestle, approximately 5 ml).

Reagents

Lysosome homogenization medium (LHM): 0.25 M sucrose, 1 mM EDTA, 20 mM Hepes–NaOH, pH 7.4

45% (w/v) Nycodenz®, 1 mM EDTA, 20 mM Hepes–NaOH, pH 7.4

Gradient solutions of 29, 26, 24 and 19% (w/v) Nycodenz®: dilute the 45% (w/v) solution with LHM.

Protocol

Keep all equipment and all solutions in ice before use and carry out all operations at 0–4°C. This protocol is designed for a liver from one adult male rat.

1. Prepare a washed light mitochondrial fraction according to steps 1–4 of *Protocol 6.5* using LHM.

2. Using a loose-fitting Dounce homogenizer resuspend the light mitochondrial pellet in 3 ml of LHM.

3. Mix 1 vol of the light mitochondrial suspension with 2 volumes 45% Nycodenz®

4. Transfer 7 ml of 19% Nycodenz® to a tube for the ultracentrifuge swinging-bucket rotor and underlayer 7 ml each of the other three gradient solutions (24, 26 and 29% Nycodenz®) and 10 ml of the light mitochondrial suspension.

5. Centrifuge at 95 000 g_{av} for 2 h and harvest the lysosomes from the 19%/24% interface.

Protocol 6.8

Rapid isolation of 'stacked' rat liver Golgi on a sucrose barrier (Morré *et al.*, 1972)

Equipment

High-speed centrifuge with swinging-bucket rotor to accommodate 30–50 ml tubes

Ultracentrifuge with swinging-bucket rotor (Beckman SW 28.1) with 17 ml tubes

Polytron homogenizer.

Reagents

Homogenization buffer (HB): 0.5 M sucrose, 1% (w/v) dextran (M_r = 225 000) in 0.05 M Tris–maleate buffer, pH 6.4

Density barrier: 1.2 M sucrose, 0.05 M Tris–maleate buffer, pH 6.4.

Protocol

Keep all equipment and all solutions in ice before use and carry out all operations at 0–4°C. This protocol is designed for a liver from one adult male rat.

1. Mince the liver finely using a razor blade and suspend in HB (approximately 10 g liver per 20 ml buffer).

2. Homogenize in a Polytron homogenizer set at 10 000 r.p.m. (setting 1) for 30–50 s.

3. Centrifuge for 15 min at 5000 g; carefully aspirate and discard the supernatant.

4. The upper (yellow–brown) portion of the bipartite pellet contains the Golgi membranes. Add 1–2 ml of HB very carefully down the wall of the slanted tube and resuspend the upper layer by *very gentle* stirring with a glass rod.

5. Avoid resuspension of the lower part of the pellet, which contains nuclei and unbroken cells.

6. Transfer the resuspended Golgi material to a new tube.

7. Adjust the concentration of the suspension with HB to 6 ml per 10 g of liver.

8. Layer over 2 volumes of the density barrier in a tube for the ultracentrifuge rotor.

9. Centrifuge at 120 000g for 30 min.

10. Remove the Golgi membranes that collect at the interface.

Note

Unstacking of the Golgi requires incubation at 4°C for 45 min with a mixture of 3 mg each of crude α-amylase Type X-A from *Aspergillus oryzae* and α-amylase Type III-A from barley.

Protocol 6.9

Fractionation of a light mitochondrial fraction in a self-generated iodixanol gradient

Equipment

Overhead electric motor, thyristor-controlled, mounted either to a wall, via a G-clamp to the bench or in a floor-standing cradle

Potter–Elvehjem homogenizer (20–30 ml: clearance approximately 0.09 mm)

High-speed centrifuge with swinging-bucket rotor to accommodate 30–50 ml tubes

Vertical rotor, near-vertical or shallow angle fixed-angle rotor for an ultracentrifuge, with tube size of 12 ml or less (e.g. Beckman VTi65.1)

Sealed tubes for the ultracentrifuge rotor

Dounce homogenizer (loose-fitting Wheaton type B pestle, approximately 30 ml)

Dounce homogenizer (loose-fitting Wheaton type B pestle, approximately 5 ml)

Gradient unloader for dense end first collection.

Reagents

Homogenization medium (HM): 0.25 M sucrose, 1 mM EDTA, 10 mM Hepes–NaOH, pH 7.4

OptiPrep™

Diluent: 0.25 M sucrose, 6 mM EDTA, 60 mM Hepes–NaOH, pH 7.4

50% (w/v) Iodixanol working stock: 5 volumes of OptiPrep plus 1 volume of diluent

25% (w/v) Iodixanol: dilute working stock with HM.

Protocol

Keep all equipment and all solutions in ice before use and carry out all operations at 0–4°C. This protocol is designed for a liver from one adult male rat.

1. Prepare a washed light mitochondrial fraction according to steps 1–4 of *Protocol 6.5* using HM described above.

2. Use two or three gentle strokes of the pestle of the Dounce homogenizer to suspend the light mitochondrial pellet in 10–12 ml of HM.

3. Mix the 50% (w/v) iodixanol stock and light mitochondrial suspension to produce a final iodixanol concentration of 17.5% (w/v).

4. Transfer to a sealed tube for the vertical, near-vertical or fixed-angle rotor allowing room to underlay the suspension with 1.0 ml of the 25% iodixanol.

5. Centrifuge at 180 000 g for 2–3 h.

6. Allow the rotor to decelerate from 1000 r.p.m. to rest either using a controlled deceleration program or without the brake.

7. Collect the gradient dense end first in approximately 1 ml fractions.

Note

The precise centrifugation conditions will depend on the sedimentation path length of the rotor (see Chapter 4). Although higher RCFs might produce appropriate density profiles in times shorter than 2–3 h, it is probably advisable to restrict the RCF to no more than approximately 200 000 g since mitochondria are very prone to disruption by hydrostatic forces.

Protocol 6.10

Isolation of plasma membrane sheets from rat liver (Hubbard *et al.*, 1983)

Equipment

Low-speed refrigerated centrifuge with swinging-bucket rotor for 50 ml tubes

Ultracentrifuge with swinging-bucket rotor (Beckman SW 28) with 38 ml tubes

Dounce homogenizer (loose-fitting Wheaton type B, 30 ml)

Nylon mesh (750 μm pore size)

Refractometer.

Reagents

Medium A: 0.25 M sucrose, 1 mM $MgCl_2$, 10 mM Tris–HCl, pH 7.4

Medium B: 2.0 M sucrose, 1 mM $MgCl_2$, 10 mM Tris–HCl, pH 7.4.

Protocol

Keep all equipment and all solutions in ice before use and carry out all operations at 0–4°C. This protocol is designed for a liver from one adult male rat.

1. Blanch the liver of an anesthetized rat by perfusing about 20 ml of Medium A. Only licensed and trained operators must carry out this procedure.

2. Rapidly excise and weigh the liver, then chop finely with scissors in a beaker on ice.

3. Suspend the mince in 30 ml of Medium A and homogenize in the Dounce homogenizer using 10 strokes of the pestle.

4. Filter the homogenate through nylon mesh, gently stirring with a glass rod to facilitate filtration.

5. Dilute the filtrate with Medium A to 5 ml g^{-1} of liver and divide between two 50-ml tubes for centrifugation at 280 g for 5 min in a swinging-bucket rotor.

6. Remove the supernatant and centrifuge this at 1500 g for 10 min.

7. Decant and discard the supernatant and resuspend the pellet in 25 ml of Medium A using the Dounce homogenizer (five strokes of the pestle).

8. Mix well with 2 volumes of Medium B and adjust the density if necessary to 1.18 g ml^{-1} (refractive index = 1.4106).

9. Divide the suspension between two tubes for the ultracentrifuge swinging-bucket rotor and fill by overlayering with about 2 ml of Medium A.

10. Centrifuge at 113 000 g for 1 h.

11. Harvest the plasma membrane sheets that band at the interface.

12. Dilute the suspension to 40 ml with HM and centrifuge at 3000 g for 10 min.

13. Resuspend the pellets in a suitable medium.

Note

The nuclei are sedimented at a lower RCF than normal to avoid loss of the plasma membrane sheets and half-filling the tubes in step 5 (shorter sedimentation path length than full tube, see Chapter 2) permits more efficient pelleting of the nuclei.

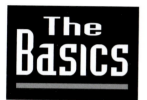

Chapter 7

Fractionation of membrane vesicles

1. The membrane compartments

This chapter is concerned with the isolation of membrane vesicles from a cell homogenate. These vesicles are derived from multiple sites.

1.1 Secretory and synthetic compartments

The major membrane compartments involved in secretion are: rough and smooth endoplasmic reticulum (RER and SER), Golgi apparatus (*cis*, median and *trans* domains), *trans*-Golgi network (TGN). In addition there are transport vesicle fractions, which shuttle between these compartments. The membrane compartments of the secretory system are also engaged in the biosynthesis and sequential post-translational modification of macromolecules, which are ultimately delivered to different subcellular destinations; there are therefore considerable sorting activities associated with some of these compartments. There are additionally retrograde circuits, which act as a conservation and control mechanism. Each membrane compartment may possess a variety of domains whose composition influences their subsequent processing.

1.2 Endocytic compartments

The situation with the endocytic process is hardly less complicated. Membrane compartments, which are involved in endocytosis, include: endocytic vesicles, coated vesicles, caveolae, primary endosomes, early endosomes, late endosomes and recycling endosomes. Different ligands are taken up at different sites on the plasma membrane and depending on the cell type these may involve relatively low-density domains of the plasma membrane such as the lipid-rich caveolae or relatively high-density clathrin-coated vesicles or some other less well-defined domain of the plasma membrane. Both clathrin-dependent and clathrin-independent endocytosis lead to the formation of smooth-surfaced primary endosomes, which then carry their cargo to tubular early endosomes that may develop into multivesicular bodies. The early endosomes act as a sorting station from which vesicles containing ligand receptors may be shunted back to the surface while the ligand proceeds, maybe via carrier vesicles, to late endosomes for ultimate delivery to lysosomes for degradation or to some other destination.

■ The system of membranes between the TGN and the surface (close to the periphery of the cell) is particularly complex and is involved in both secretory and endocytic processes, and is also a major site of sorting. For example, shuttling of the glucose-transport protein GLUT4 to and from the cell surface, in response to nutritional requirements, clearly involves various elements of both the TGN and the endocytic system.

1.3   The plasma membrane

The third type of membrane (the destination and source of the two processes described above) is the plasma membrane, which may be present in the homogenate either as vesicles or as sheets. Sheets or large fragments of plasma membrane are normally only released from specific domains of cells in organized tissues such as the liver, kidney or intestinal mucosa. On the other hand, the plasma membrane from cultured cells (even if these are functionally polarized) and from some domains of cells from organized tissues is always released as vesicles.

Caco-2 and MDCK cells have become very popular for studying how the cell sorts proteins destined for insertion into specific domains. Protein sorting to the different domains of the plasma membrane can occur either within the TGN prior to directed transfer to the domains or, if there is no sorting at this intracellular level, there could be a reallocation of specific proteins from one domain of the plasma membrane to another by transcytosis. Separation of these plasma membrane domains is clearly a prerequisite for studies into these processes.

■   The use of these polarized cultured cells is usually carried as monolayers grown in special chambers which allow defined access to both the basolateral and apical surfaces.

2.   Density and size of membrane vesicles

The density and size of membrane vesicles depends on cell type and the fractionation protocol, thus only a few general comments are useful. In sucrose their density varies $1.06–1.15 \, \mathrm{g \, ml^{-1}}$, except for rough ER ($1.18–1.23 \, \mathrm{g \, ml^{-1}}$). Vesicles are normally in the range 0.05–0.4 µm in diameter, although some plasma membrane vesicles may be up to 1.0 µm. As a general rule, the vesicles of the secretory system from the RER to the TGN decrease in density in that order. Like most of the large organelles (see Chapter 6) membrane vesicles are also osmotically active so they too lose water to hyperosmotic sucrose gradients. Nevertheless, there are numerous protocols based on sucrose and other media and the choice of gradient medium has to be considered on a case-by-case basis.

■   In secretory cells, the composition of the enclosed compartment of membrane vesicles, for example from the endoplasmic reticulum (ER) and Golgi, will influence their density and depend on the nature of the product the cells are secreting. Thus vesicles containing, for example, very low-density lipoproteins will be considerably lighter than those which contain a proteoglycan.

Of the major compartments that are common to the secretory and synthetic pathways it is probably only the densest (RER) and lightest (Golgi) which can be isolated simply and in a relatively pure form (*Protocols 7.1* and *7.3*, respectively), although a number of gradient systems can effectively separate the RER, SER and Golgi membranes and possibly the plasma membrane (*Protocol 7.6*). Generally speaking, the vesicles are separated on the basis of density rather than size, although the peripheral membrane compartments which involve the TGN and parts of the endocytic system, for example those responsible for the regulation of the GLUT4 glucose transporter, have such a similar density in sucrose gradients that only rate-zonal centrifugation (sedimentation velocity) can provide a means of analyzing this process (see Sections 3.3 and 8.2).

■ In endocytosis, the density of vesicles may reflect the nature of the ligand which is being taken up by the cells. Vesicles containing transferrin (an iron-containing protein), for example, are likely to be denser than those containing low-density lipoprotein.

There is also a pronounced tendency for the membrane compartments associated with endocytosis (particularly the early to late endosome phase) to exhibit a progressive increase in size, so that rate-zonal gradients may be effective for analyzing this process.

The plasma membrane is often the lightest membrane in isoosmotic gradients; this may be related to the fact that the size of plasma membrane vesicles tends to be rather larger than those from other sites, that is, they contain a larger aqueous compartment. The situation is complicated, however, by the existence of domains and the association of noncovalently-bound macromolecules.

■ Some plasma membrane domains may be of a very low density such as the lipid-rich caveolae and lipid rafts of epithelial and endothelial cells (but which may be present in a modified form in other types of cell).
■ Other plasma membrane domains may be dense due to association either on the outer surface with an extensive carbohydrate-rich coat or on the cytoplasmic surface with protein-rich structures such as clathrin coats (coated pits) or elements of the cytoskeleton.
■ The presence of an extensive cytoskeleton may also determine how the plasma membrane behaves under homogenization.

The apical domain from polarized cultured cells (e.g. MDCK and Caco-2) is normally a brush-border type membrane, which may be rendered denser by association with the proteins of a cytoskeleton. Only in the case of an organized tissue, however, such as rat liver, may domains behave differentially in the homogenization process to yield large sheets or small vesicles.

3. Separation strategies

3.1 The microsomal fraction

There are countless different types of gradient that have been used for studying specific vesicle fractions that form part of the secretory, synthetic or endocytic systems. These are often tailored to a particular cell type or macromolecular processing and clearly this text cannot survey these comprehensively. Nevertheless there are a few widely used protocols for studying the principal compartments, which are given at the end of the chapter

The vesicles described in Sections 1 and 2 are components of the microsomal fraction, which, in the case of an organized tissue such as liver, are normally resolved from a 100 000 g microsomal fraction or from a post-light mitochondrial supernatant. Parenchymal liver cells have large complements of other denser and more rapidly sedimenting organelles which need to be removed prior to carrying out gradient separation of the vesicle fraction. In the case of cultured cells, however, it is often only necessary to remove the nuclei from the homogenate and the use of a post-nuclear supernatant as the gradient input is very common. Moreover, the inclusion of a differential centrifugation step at 12–15 000 g to remove the larger organelles (mitochondria, lysosomes, etc.) often leads to a significant loss of membrane vesicles into this pellet. This is often exacerbated by the tendency of the 12 000–15 000 g pellet from cultured cells to be difficult to disaggregate, thus making recovery of any vesicles by pellet washing inefficient.

3.2 Density-gradient fractionation

The methods used to fractionate the vesicles often rely on the standard technology of discontinuous and continuous gradients using both buoyant-density and rate-zonal modes. Although there are a number of standard techniques for separating some of the major compartments, protocols are likely to require customization to the particular separation problem.

Except when it is required to isolate a specific membrane compartment for detailed functional studies, it is often not necessary for the gradient to separate pure populations of the various compartments. Indeed, because of the heterogeneity within each compartment and the continuous nature of the secretory, synthetic and endocytic processes, it is unlikely that any gradient would be able to resolve as distinct bands, for example, the *cis-*, median and *trans*-domains of the Golgi or ER-Golgi intermediate vesicles from the ER and *cis*-Golgi. So long as there is some reproducible and distinctive pattern in the gradient of markers for each of the compartments, then such gradients can be used to study the processing of macromolecules as they pass through these systems.

Sometimes, however, it is possible to use some particular characteristic of the membrane vesicle, either some intrinsic lipid or protein component of the membrane itself or a macromolecule that is within the vesicle as a result of a secretory or endocytic process, to target that vesicle with some sort of probe. That probe may result in modulation of its density (immunoaffinity and density perturbation techniques) and consequently permit it to be separated more specifically from the bulk of the untagged vesicles. In other situations, an enclosed macromolecule, which can be tagged by, for example by radio-labeling, is used merely to identify the vesicle rather than to aid its purification.

3.3 Gradient media for vesicle fractionation

Most of the protocols for the isolation and analysis of the membrane compartments of the secretory, synthetic and endocytic pathways use sucrose as a gradient medium. Its cheapness and the huge literature on the use of sucrose gradients make this a first choice for many workers. As with all work with sucrose, significant disadvantages stem from the high osmolarity and viscosity of its gradient. Any opportunity to resolve vesicles on the basis of their native density (membrane plus water compartment) or size is thus compromised and the high viscosity means that small membrane vesicles need long run times in order to achieve equilibrium density banding. Sucrose/D_2O gradients were introduced to reduce the viscosity problem while maintaining the required density range (see Chapter 3 and Section 8.1).

Iodinated density-gradient media (metrizamide, Nycodenz® and iodix-anol) have provided a number of alternative methodologies, which intro-duce some important advantages. Notably, these are the ability to use an isoosmotic density gradient in which to fractionate endocytic compart-ments on the basis of size (Section 9.2) and the use of iodixanol in a self-generating mode (Sections 8.3 and 9.3) to facilitate sample handling and provide the necessary reproducibility of gradient-density profiles when using gradients in an analytical mode to study secretion and endocytosis. Percoll® has also been used to fractionate membrane vesicles but it has not generally found a wide application in this area because the centrifugation conditions required to band the vesicles are liable to cause significant sed-imentation of the colloidal particles; thus it is difficult to obtain density profiles which are not very shallow at the top and very steep at the bottom.

An excellent example of the comparison of sucrose and iodixanol strat-egies comes from the analysis of the translocation of the GLUT4 glucose trans-porter through the peripheral membrane compartments of adipocytes. In sucrose gradients, density differences between the various compartments are too small to analyze and the strategy is to fractionate low density membrane vesicles by sedimentation velocity (see Section 8.2) through pre-formed linear 10–30% sucrose gradients (e.g. Zhou et al., 2000). Even though the osmotic gradient probably leads to progressive shrinkage of the vesicles, this effect may either be ameliorated by the short centrifugation time (<1 h) or maybe differ-ent vesicles respond in different ways. In iodixanol on the other hand the membrane vesicle fraction can be very effectively resolved on the basis of density in an isoosmotic self-generated gradient using a 14% iodixanol start-ing concentration (Hashiramoto and James, 2000). Whether the density of the vesicles is dictated principally by the size of the enclosed water space or by some other compositional parameter is not clear. The analysis of these gradients is too complex to be presented in further detail in this text and the reader should consult the two references for further information.

Although recent applications of iodixanol may make analytical work on the vesicles associated with secretion and endocytosis much simpler, through the use of self-generated gradients (Sections 8.3 and 9.3), there is no general observation that one medium is much better than another in all situations.

The following sections consider techniques for the isolation of ER (Section 4), Golgi membranes (Section 5) and plasma membrane (Section 6). Section 7 is concerned broadly with the use an applications of density perturbation, while Sections 8 and 9 address the use of analytical techniques for studying secretion and endocytosis, respectively.

4. Endoplasmic reticulum

Vesicles of the RER and SER make up the bulk of the microsomal fraction. which sediments predominantly at about 100 000 g for 30–40 min. Frac-tionation of the microsomes is normally carried out using this 100 000 g pellet, but the light mitochondrial supernatant is an alternative starting material. Simple bulk separation of SER and RER from rat liver can be achieved on a discontinuous CsCl-containing sucrose gradient using the light mitochondrial fraction of a tissue homogenate. The Cs^+ ions seem to act by binding preferentially to the RER, thus decreasing their surface negative charge, thereby allowing them to aggregate and raising their rate of sedimentation through a dense barrier (*Protocol 7.1*). The separation is thus partly on the basis of density and partly on the basis of sedimentation velocity.

An alternative continuous gradient described in *Protocol 7.2* has the potential for identifying subfractions of the ER, which may be useful in analyzing a secretory or synthetic process. This is not possible in the sucrose–CsCl barrier system. It also serves to highlight (i) a contamination problem and (ii) a solution to this problem, which is, in effect, one of the earliest examples of the use of density perturbation. The RER tends be contaminated with peroxisome cores, which have overlapping densities: the solution is to strip the ribosomes from the RER chemically using pyrophosphate and thus make the membrane vesicles lighter, after they have first been separated from the smooth membrane fraction.

5. Golgi membranes

As with the preparation of intact Golgi stacks and Golgi tubules (Chapter 6), Golgi vesicles are routinely isolated as a low-density fraction by banding them at the upper interface of a layer of sucrose, below which most of the other membranes either band or pellet. This approach is commonly used with a whole homogenate or a post-nuclear supernatant from cultured cells but a light mitochondrial supernatant or microsomal fraction may also be used. A concentration of approximately 40% (w/v) sucrose (approximately $\rho = 1.15$ g ml^{-1}) is normally effective (Balch *et al.*, 1984) for floating the Golgi away from other membranes; occasionally a lower density (approximately $\rho = 1.11$ g ml^{-1}) may be used (see *Protocol 7.3*). In the case of rat liver, sometimes both are used to obtain light and heavy fractions of Golgi – a light and a heavy fraction (Sztul *et al.*, 1985).

This protocol can be used in conjunction with others for the fractionation of the SER and RER if the Golgi membranes are prepared from a light mitochondrial supernatant (or total microsomal fraction). The vesicles of the ER remaining in the load zone of the gradient (*Protocol 7.3*) may be subsequently resolved in the sucrose–CsCl barrier system (*Protocol 7.1*) or in a linear sucrose gradient (*Protocol 7.2*). For an example of this approach, see Sztul *et al.* (1985) and Macintyre (1992).

Partial separation of the *cis*-, medial- and *trans*-domains of the Golgi can be obtained in some sucrose gradients, but the overlapping nature of their densities considerably limits their resolution. It has also been observed that partial separation can only be achieved if long periods of centrifugation (20 h) are allowed for the membranes to reach 'apparent equilibrium' (Dunphy and Rothman, 1983).

6. Plasma membrane and membrane domains

The isolation of sheets of plasma membrane from the nuclear pellet of a rat liver homogenate is described in Chapter 6. This short section is devoted exclusively to plasma membrane domain methods, while Section 7 is concerned with methods that are relevant to plasma membrane vesicles and other vesicles.

6.1 From membrane particles containing more than one domain

If an isolated membrane fraction contains two domains that are both functionally and compositionally distinct, then the potential exists for separation of these domains by density-gradient centrifugation after they have
been cleaved by some sort of shearing force. Often this shearing force is sonication but vigorous liquid shear might be an alternative. Sonication is used,
for example, to separate the contiguous and bile canalicular membrane
domains, which are parts of the plasma membrane sheets (Chapter 6).
Because the contiguous domain is associated with protein-rich desmosomes,
this domain is relatively dense and can be separated from the lighter bile
canalicular membrane in a sucrose gradient (Scott et al., 1992). Although
Hubbard et al. (1983) used a continuous linear sucrose gradient (0.46–1.42
M) a narrow range discontinuous gradient of 35, 39 and 44% (w/v) sucrose
at 196 000 g_{av} for 3 h (Meier et al., 1984) seems quite satisfactory. The
canalicular membrane bands mainly at the sample/gradient interface and
the basolateral (contiguous) domain bands at the 39/44% interface.

In the last 8–10 years, two specialized domains of the plasma membrane of
epithelial and endothelial cells have received considerable research attention:
caveolae and lipid rafts. They are both lipid-rich domains of the plasma membrane and they are both involved in some important aspects of intracellular
signaling and metabolic control. Caveolae can also be released from plasma
membrane preparations by sonication and because of their lipid-rich nature
they are relatively light. After sonication, isoosmotic gradients of iodixanol are
used to separate the caveolae from the denser areas of the plasma membrane
(Uittenbogaard et al., 1998).

6.2 Selective solubilization

Another approach to the separation of a lipid-rich domain is a commonly
used strategy for lipid rafts. The high level of sphingolipid and cholesterol in
this domain makes it relatively insensitive to solubilization by the nonionic
detergent Triton X-100. In this case no prior purification of a plasma membrane fraction is necessary. Since all of the membranes of the cell (with the
exception of the nuclear membrane) are susceptible to nonionic detergents,
a post-nuclear supernatant from the cell homogenate is adjusted to 1%
Triton X-100 and 40% iodixanol. This is layered beneath a discontinuous
gradient of 0, 20, 25, 30 and 35% (w/v) iodixanol (also containing the
detergent) and during centrifugation the lipid rafts float to the top of the
20% iodixanol layer. The solubilized membrane proteins are dense and
therefore remain in the load zone (Lafont et al., 1999).

6.3 Separation of plasma membrane domains from polarized
cells

Ellis et al. (1992) devised a density-gradient method for isolating the two
plasma membrane domains from Caco-2 cells grown on permeable filter
supports which is described in a flow chart (*Figure 7.1*)

- ■ Differential precipitation. This protocol is noteworthy for the use of
  10 mM Mg^{2+} to remove membranes that might otherwise contaminate
  the products of interest. Bivalent cations (either Ca^{2+} or Mg^{2+}) can be
  used to remove selectively less negatively charged membranes.

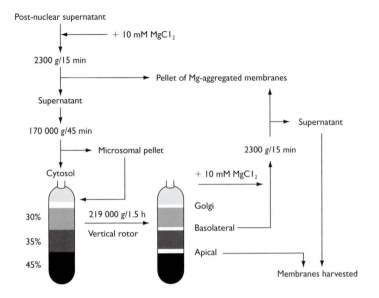

Figure 7.1

Fractionation of Caco-2 cell plasma membrane domains. Adapted from Ellis et al. (1992).

7.   Isolation of vesicular membranes by density perturbation

Because many vesicles derived from plasma membrane domains and also from other compartments of the secretory and endocytic systems types have overlapping densities, their isolation on a preparative basis often requires some form of density-perturbation technique to enhance selectively the density of a particular vesicle type. The strategy is to use some compositional or functional parameter that is characteristic of a certain type of membrane vesicle to permit the selective binding of a molecule or particle that causes a density enhancement of that vesicle. In this manner its separation from other vesicles not bearing this parameter or from vesicles whose orientation does not allow binding of the molecule or particle is achieved.

7.1   Immunoaffinity

This success of this strategy relies on the fact that during homogenization of cells (or tissues), vesicles formed from the plasma membrane tend to retain their correct orientation, that is, the surface that is exposed to the liquid environment *in vitro* is the same as the surface that is exposed to the extracellular environment *in vivo* (*Figure 7.2*). The strategy can also be used for intracellular membranes and it is equally important that the vesicles formed from the ER, Golgi, *et cetera* also retain their normal orientation, that is, the face exposed to the cytosol *in vivo* is exposed to the liquid environment *in vitro*. The cisternal contents of the tubular membrane systems, which are sequestered away from the cytosol *in vivo*, are similarly sequestered away from the liquid environment *in vitro* (*Figure 7.2*).

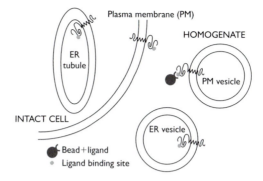

Figure 7.2

Preferential binding of ligand to exposed sites on plasma membrane vesicles. The figure shows a bead-bound ligand binding to the ligand binding site of an integral protein of plasma membrane vesicles. In endoplasmic reticulum (ER) vesicles the ligand binding site is sequestered within the vesicle and not available to the bead-ligand (for more information see text).

Proteins (or glycoproteins) synthesized and modified within the cisternae of the cytoplasmic membrane systems are ultimately expressed at the external surface of the plasma membrane or plasma membrane domain; thus, any ligand (often an antibody) to the extracellular polypeptide sequence of an integral protein can only bind to a plasma membrane vesicle containing this protein (*Figure 7.2*). Only an antibody to the original cytoplasmic polypeptide tail of an integral protein will bind selectively to a vesicle from the intracellular membranes. If the antibody is bound a dense bead, then the appropriate vesicles will be rendered considerably denser. The process is called immunoaffinity isolation (Howell *et al.*, 1988).

The method requires either a secondary antibody or protein A to act as a bridge between the bead and the probing primary antibody in order to avoid any steric hindrance to bead binding. The following beads types have been used:

- derivatized cellulose (diazocellulose) used by Luzio and Richardson (1993) for isolation of cholinergic nerve terminals;
- commercially available Protein A-Sepharose (Sztul *et al.*, 1985);
- intact (protein A-bearing) *Staphylococcus aureus* (Hubbard *et al.*, 1988).

Using an antibody to the cytoplasmic tail of a number of cell surface receptors, Hubbard *et al.* (1988) isolated intracellular pools of these receptors and were able to distinguish them from other membranes.

Practical notes

- The secondary antibody (immunoglobulin G; IgG) can be linked by hydrophobic interaction to a bead, but it is generally considered preferable to link it covalently.
- It is recommended that at least a two-fold excess of primary antibody should be used for binding to the IgG-bead. This coupling is routinely carried out overnight just prior to use.
- Alternatively the primary antibody can be reacted with the unpurified membrane suspension rather than with the IgG-bead. Better results are

reported, for example, if the primary antibody is reacted first with the membranes rather than with the *S. aureus* (Hubbard *et al.*, 1988). In this case, unreacted antibody must be removed by centrifugation and washing or by centrifuging through a density barrier prior to addition of the IgG-bead.

A typical method for the isolation of the sinusoidal domain from hepatocytes is given in *Protocol 7.4*. It uses the polymeric immunoglobulin A (IgA) receptor (sometimes called the secretory component) as the domain-specific antigen.

7.2   Lectin–gold

An alternative probe, which can be bound selectively to the plasma membrane, is a lectin such as wheat-germ agglutinin (WGA). Lectins bind to specific carbohydrate residues of membrane integral proteins. As these are only exposed to the external medium on vesicles derived from the plasma membrane (and not those derived from intracellular membranes), a probe of WGA bound to dense colloidal gold will effectively raise the density only of the plasma membrane vesicles. This approach was developed by Gupta and Tartakoff (1989) for separating Golgi membranes from plasma membrane as, in their native form, these tend to overlap in density gradients, particularly of sucrose.

■   The sugar specificity of WGA is *N*-acetylglucosamine, so sucrose will not compete for the binding site, but metrizamide will (metrizamide contains an *N*-acetylglucosamine residue).

To improve the cross-linking of WGA to the gold colloid, Gupta and Tartakoff (1989) increased its molecular size by linking it covalently to bovine serum albumin (BSA).

■   Intact cells are incubated with the lectin–BSA–gold for 30–60 min at 4°C, then washed to remove excess reagent. After homogenization of the cells, the suspension is adjusted to 0.25 M with respect to sucrose and fractionated in a 20–40% sucrose gradient. Compared to untreated cells, plasma membrane markers are shifted to the bottom of the gradient while Golgi markers are unaffected.

7.3   Horseradish peroxidase

A commonly used method for resolving endosomes from Golgi fractions depends on the ability to modulate the density of the endosomes once they have taken up a horseradish peroxidase (HRP)-linked ligand (Courtoy *et al.*, 1984). In the presence of hydrogen peroxide, the enzyme oxidizes 3,3'-diaminobenzidine (DAB) and it is this reaction which is considered responsible for the resulting raised density of the endosomes.

Any suitable ligand can be chosen and linked to HRP and presented to either isolated cells or an intact tissue. Courtoy *et al.* (1984) used neogalactosylalbumin as the ligand coupled to HRP, which was injected into rats intravenously (1 µg g^{-1} of bodyweight) for 10 min prior to liver perfusion, excision and homogenization.

■ A crude Golgi/endosome fraction is incubated in 5 mM DAB, with or without (as control) 11 mM H_2O_2 at 25°C for 15–30 min. The membrane suspension is then centrifuged through a suitable sucrose gradient (e.g. ρ = 1.1–1.3 g ml^{-1}) at 240 000 g for 100 min. The density of the endosomes is shifted from 1.13 to 1.21 g ml^{-1}.

7.4 Digitonin

The ability of digitonin to form a stable covalent complex with cholesterol has also been used to density-perturb those membranes (e.g. plasma membrane and Golgi membranes) which are rich in this lipid (Amar-Costesec *et al.*, 1974).

Digitonin (0.235%, w/v) is added drop-wise to membranes suspended in 0.25 M sucrose with continuous stirring (final digitonin concentration = 0.17%). After standing at 0°C for 15 min excess soluble digitonin is removed by dilution with buffer and pelleting before recentrifuging the membranes through a suitable gradient. The cholesterol:phospholipid molar ratio of the ER is about 0.1, considerably lower than that of the plasma membrane (up to 1.0) and Golgi membranes (approximately 0.5). In sucrose gradients the mean density of endoplasmic reticulum is unaffected, while that of the plasma membrane is shifted by about 0.03 g ml^{-1}, and that of Golgi membranes is shifted by 0.015 g ml^{-1} (Amar-Costesec *et al.*, 1974).

8. Analytical gradients (secretion)

There is a vast literature on the use of a variety of sucrose gradients to study both the secretory and endocytic processes, and for reviews of these see, respectively, Graham (1997) and Gjøen *et al.* (1997). Only a few illustrative examples can be given here.

8.1 Sucrose equilibrium density gradients

One of the most successful strategies for the study of various aspects of the secretory process is the sucrose–D_2O gradient system (*Protocol 7.5*) devised by Lodish *et al.* (1987), which was designed primarily to study the transfer of proteins from the rough endoplasmic reticulum to the *cis*-Golgi. The gradient showed that this transfer involved a low-density vesicle quite distinct from its source and destination membranes. The use of D_2O as a solvent is a means of increasing the density of sucrose gradients without increasing their viscosity (see Chapter 3), thus the method also has the advantage of using relatively low g-forces and short centrifugation times (160 000 g for 3 h). The resolution of the gradient is enhanced by collection of the gradients in small fraction volumes (12 ml gradients in 32 fractions). Low-density ER–Golgi intermediates band in the region 12.5–17.5% sucrose, while the ER itself bands around 22% sucrose. The gradients are also capable of a high degree of resolution of ER–Golgi–TGN events (Miller *et al.*, 1992) and subfractionation of the Golgi membranes (Moore and Spiro, 1992).

8.2 Sucrose velocity gradients

Sucrose equilibrium density gradients on their own are rather less successful at resolving the vesicles post-Golgi events. Tooze and Huttner (1990) used a sedimentation velocity gradient, followed by a second equilibrium density gradient to fractionate TGN vesicle and post-TGN vesicles (*Protocol 7.6*). The second sucrose gradient used by Tooze and Hunter (1990) was extremely steep (approximately $\rho = 1.06–1.25$ g ml^{-1}) and a shallower gradient or use of an iodinated density-gradient medium (see Section 8.3) may be more suitable. A sucrose velocity gradient covering the range $\rho = 1.04–1.14$ g ml^{-1} seems to have a broad applicability to a study of post-TGN to plasma membrane events and similar gradients have been popular for analyzing the important translocation of glucose transporter (GLUT4) vesicles from the periphery of the cell to the cell surface (Zhou *et al.*, 2000). The main variable is the centrifugation time, which may be as low as 15 min (Tooze and Huttner, 1990) and as high as 55 min (Zhou *et al.*, 2000) and will depend on the size of the vesicles of interest.

8.3   Iodixanol equilibrium density gradients

Simultaneous isolation of the Golgi, SER and RER is probably best accomplished in isoosmotic gradients of iodixanol: either pre-formed continuous gradients covering the range 4–26% (w/v) iodixanol ($\rho = 1.05–1.56$ g ml^{-1}) in a swinging-bucket rotor at 200 000 g for approximately 2–3 h (Yang *et al.*, 1997; Zhang *et al.*, 1998), or the separation can be carried out in a self-generated gradient. The original self-generated method – centrifuging a microsome fraction in 20% (w/v) iodixanol in a vertical rotor (Cartwright *et al.*, 1997) was designed primarily for analyzing the SER and RER. This was subsequently developed to include resolution of the Golgi using a starting configuration of equal volumes of 15 and 20% (w/v) iodixanol (*Protocol 7.7*). *Figure 7.3* shows that the Golgi (galactosyl transferase) bands at the top of the gradient, with the NADPH-cytochrome *c* reductase showing two bands – the lower-density band contains no RNA (SER), while the denser one exhibits an RNA content which increases towards the bottom of the gradient (RER). The method minimizes the number of steps and the use of vertical rotors makes the procedure very efficient (Plonné *et al.*, 1999).

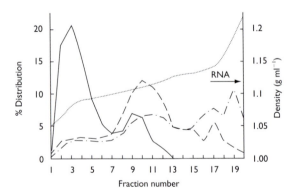

Figure 7.3

Fractionation of hepatocyte microsomes in a self-generated gradient of iodixanol: % distribution of membrane markers. The method is described in Protocol 7.7; *density (·······), protein (— ·), NADPH-cytochrome c-reductase (endoplasmic reticulum; ER – –), UDP-galactose galactosyltransferase (Golgi ——). RNA (an RER marker) is found in the region shown by the arrow. Data adapted from Plonné et al. (1999)* Anal Biochem. **276***: 88–96.*

Iodinated density-gradient media also offer a significant improvement in resolution of Golgi domains. A discontinuous gradient of Nycodenz® or iodixanol (10, 15, 20, 25 and 30%, w/v) centrifuged at 250 000 g for 4 h can resolve different functional activities of the Golgi (galactosyl transferase and O-sulfotransferase) and simultaneously, vesicles responsible for transport of proteoglycans to the surface (Graham and Winterbourne, 1988).

9   Analytical gradients (endocytosis)

9.1 Operational strategies

Monolayer cells

A common approach to the study of endocytosis is firstly to incubate cells with the ligand of choice (often radiolabeled) at 0°C. After ligand binding has occurred, the cell monolayer is washed several times at 0°C to remove any unbound ligand and the temperature is raised to 37°C for varying times to allow internalization to proceed, after which the cells are again rapidly cooled to 0°C. At the zero time and each successive timepoint the cells are homogenized and fractionated in a density gradient (*Figure 7.4*).

At 0°C endocytosis is arrested and so at zero time any membrane fraction in a gradient that contains the radiolabel is operationally identified as plasma membrane. Furthermore, essentially all of the plasma membrane vesicles formed during homogenization of the cells retain their original orientation (i.e. the outer face of the vesicle is the extracellular face of the intact

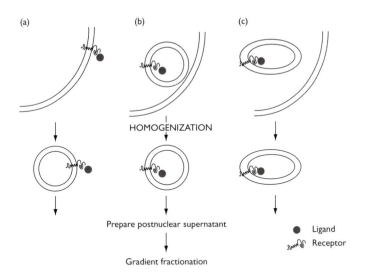

Figure 7.4

Pulse-chase strategy for studying uptake of a ligand by endocytosis in cultured cells. (a) The radiolabeled ligand is allowed to bind to its receptor (an integral glycoprotein) on the cell surface at 0°C; endocytosis is arrested and the only vesicles bearing the radiolabel are from the plasma membrane. (b) After washing to remove unbound ligand, the cells are returned to 37°C and the ligand is taken up by endocytosis. The ligand appears in a primary endosome. (c) At a later time the ligand appears in others particles such as early endosomes (see Section 1.2 for more details). As the particles described in (a–c) have different densities and sizes, by cooling the cells to 0°C, homogenizing and gradient fractionation at different time intervals the process can be analyzed (see Figures 7.5–7.8).

membrane). Thus only the ligand on plasma membrane vesicles is available to *in vitro* manipulation either by enzymic degradation or destabilization of the ligand-receptor link (e.g. in the case of the asialoglycoprotein receptor by EDTA). This is not the case with any endocytic compartment (*Figure 7.4*).

Perfused liver

This system is not so readily or precisely manipulated as the cell culture system, but it is closer to the *in vivo* situation. The exposed organ from an anesthetized animal is made part of continuous perfusion system. The pumped fluid (which is normally human blood) in the closed system is maintained at 37°C and passes over a gas-exchange device so that oxygenated blood is delivered to the liver. This continuous system can be interrupted to operate as a single pass such that a pulse of labeled ligand can be injected into the fluid flow and the effluent from the liver collected. At each time point the warmed oxygenated fluid is replaced by ice-cold homogenization medium and the liver rapidly excised and processed.

9.2   Sedimentation velocity gradients

Iodinated density-gradient media are a popular choice for these separations. A post-nuclear supernatant is loaded on to a 0–35% Nycodenz® (or iodixanol) gradient and centrifuged at 85 000 g for 45 min (Kindberg *et al.*, 1984). *Figure 7.5* shows the distribution of ^{125}I-asiaiofetuin on Nycodenz® gradients after internalization during incubation of a rat liver hepatocytes for different times. After 1 min, only a small amount of the ligand has been internalized and is associated with slowly sedimenting particles. With increasing times, more ligand becomes internalized and the distribution of radiolabel demonstrates that the endocytic structures containing the ligand increase their sedimentation rate (Kindberg *et al.*, 1984).

Rate-zonal Nycodenz® gradients can also identify pre-lysosomal and lysosomal compartments in the 1.14–1.16 g ml^{-1} density region (Malaba *et al.*, 1995).

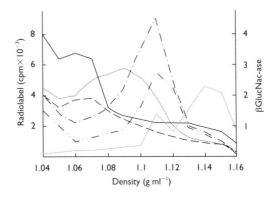

Figure 7.5

Rate-zonal analysis of endocytosis in 0–35% Nycodenz® gradients: distribution of radiolabel. The uptake of ^{125}I-labeled asialofetuin by hepatocytes was studied using a pulse-chase strategy (see Figure 7.4). At each time point a post-nuclear supernatant from an homogenate was layered on a gradient and centrifuged at 85 000 g for 45 min (see text for further details). (——) 0.5 min, (– –) 1 min, (··········) 2.5 min, (— ·) 15 min, (— ··) 30 min, (——) β-N acetylglucosaminidase (a lysosome marker). Data adapted from Kindberg et al. (1984) Anal. Biochem. 142: 455–462, with kind permission of the authors and Academic Press.

9.3   Buoyant (equilibrium) density

Continuous gradients prepared from Optiprep™ can separate early and recycling endosomes (*Figure 7.6*): a post-nuclear supernatant is layered on to a
5–20% or 10–20% iodixanol gradient and centrifuged at 90 000 g_{av} for 18 h
in a 13–14 ml swinging-bucket rotor (Sheff *et al.*, 1999) The gradient is also
able to resolve plasma membrane and lysosomes. Long centrifugation times
ensure that all the vesicles in a top-loaded sample reach their buoyant
density, but it is important not to use significantly higher relative centrifugal
fields (RCFs) since the sedimentation of iodixanol will distort the pre-
formed gradient, particularly at the bottom of the tube.

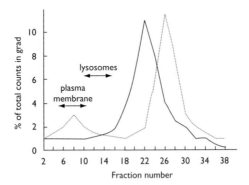

Figure 7.6

Buoyant density analysis of endocytosis in 5–20% iodixanol gradients: distribution of ligand.
The uptake of transferrin by MDCK cells was studied by a pulse-chase strategy (see Figure
7.4). At different times a post-nuclear supernatant from an homogenate was layered on a gra-
dient and centrifuged at 95 000 g for 18–20 h (see text for details). The gradient was
unloaded low-density end first; (⋯⋯) 2.5 min, (——) 25 min. The position in the gradient
of plasma membrane and lysosomes is indicated by the arrows. Data adapted from Sheff et al.
*(1999) J. Cell Biol. **145**: 123–129, with kind permission of the authors and The Rockefeller*
Press.

Self-generated gradients

The flow chart that is *Figure 7.7* illustrates a different approach to the analysis of the endocytic process. By using OptiPrep™ in a self-generated mode,

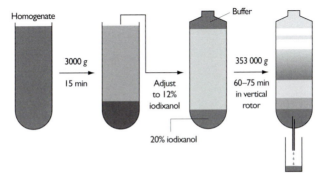

Figure 7.7

Strategy for analyzing endocytosis by buoyant density in self-generated iodixanol gradients.

quite large volumes of a post-nuclear (or post-heavy mitochondrial) supernatant can be simply mixed with the medium to a suitable iodixanol
starting concentration and centrifuged for 1–3 h in a vertical or near-vertical
rotor at approximately 350 000 g.

■   By changing the centrifugation conditions, the density profile of the
     gradient can be easily modulated for improved resolution of specific
     membrane vesicles.

Figure 7.8 shows the analysis of endocytosis using the perfused rat liver
method (Billington *et al.*, 1998). The example given uses ^{99m}Tc-labeled neogalactosylalbumin as the ligand and following a 1-min pulse of the ligand,
perfusion with unlabeled medium is continued for chase times of 1–20 min.
The figure shows that these gradients can resolve dense clathrin-coated
vesicles (1–2-min chase), light endosomes (10-min chase) and lysosomes
(20-min chase).

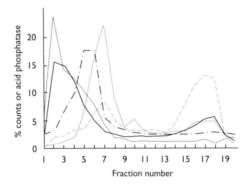

Figure 7.8

*Buoyant density analysis of endocytosis of radiolabeled neogalactosyl albumin by rat liver in
self-generated 12.5% iodixanol gradients: distribution of radiolabel. At different times the
liver was homogenized and analyzed according to* Figure 7.7. *The gradient was unloaded
dense-end first: (— ·) 1 min, (——) 2 min, (- - -) 10 min, (——) 20 min, (·········) acid phosphatase (lysosomes). Clathrin is detected in fractions 3–9. Data adapted from Billington* et al.
(1998) Anal. Biochem. *258: 251–258, with kind permission of Academic Press.*

References

Amar-Costesec, A., Wibo, M., Thinès-Sempoux, D., Beaufay, H. and Berthet, J.
(1974) Analytical study of microsomes and isolated subcellular membranes
from rat liver. IV Biochemical, physical and morphological modification of
microsomal components induced by digitonin, EDTA and pyrophosphate. *J. Cell
Biol.* **62:** 717–745.

Amar-Costesec, A., Godelaine, D. and Hortsch, M. (1988). Purification of membranes enriched in rough endoplasmic reticulum domain by a density pertur-
bant. In: *Cell Free Analysis of Membrane Traffic* (ed. D. J. Morré, K. E. Howell,
G. M. C. Cook and W. H. Evans). Alan R Liss Inc., New York, pp. 211–225.

Balch, W. E., Dunphy, W. G., Braell, W. A. and Rothman, J. E. (1984)
Reconsitution of the transport of protein between successive compartments of
the Golgi measured by the coupled incorporation of N-acetylglucosamine. *Cell*
39: 405–416.

Bergstrand, A. and Dallner, G. (1969) Isolation of rough and smooth microsomes
from rat liver by means of a commercially available centrifuge. *Anal. Biochem.*
29: 351–356.

Billington, D., Maltby, P.J., Jackson, A.P. and Graham, J.M. (1998) Dissection of hepatic receptor-mediated endocytic pathways using self-generated gradients of iodixanol (OptiPrep). *Anal. Biochem.* **258**: 251–258.

Cartwright, I.J., Higgins, J.A., Wilkinson, J., Bellavia, S., Kendrick, J.S. and Graham, J.M. (1997) Investigation of the role of lipids in the assembly of very low density lipoproteins in rabbit hepatocytes. *J. Lipid Res.* **38**: 531–545.

Courtoy, P.J., Quintart, J., and Baudhuin, P. (1984) Shift of equilibrium density induced by 3,3'-diaminobenzidine cytochemistry: a new procedure for the analysis of peroxidase containing organelles. *J. Cell Biol.* **98**: 870–876.

Dunphy, W.G. and Rothman, J.E. (1983) Compartmentation of Asn-linked oligosaccharide processing in the Golgi apparatus. *J. Cell Biol.* **97**: 270–275.

Ellis, J.A., Jackman, M.R. and M.R. and Luzio, J.P. (1992) the post-synthetic sorting of endogenous membrane proteins examined by the simultaneous purification of apical and basolateral plasma membrane fractions from Caco-2 cells. *Biohem. J.* **283**: 553–560.

Gjøen, T., Berg, T.O. and Berg, T. (1997) Lysosomes and endocytosis. In: *Subcellular Fractionation – A Practical Approach* (eds J.M. Graham and D. Rickwood). IRL Press at Oxford University Press, Oxford, pp. 169–203.

Graham, J.M. (1997) The membranes of the secretory and exocytic pathways. In: *Subcellular Fractionation – A Practical Approach* (eds J.M. Graham and D. Rickwood). IRL Press at Oxford University Press, Oxford, pp. 205–241.

Graham, J.M. and Winterbourne, D.J. (1988) Subcellular localization of the sulphation reaction of heparan sulphate synthesis and transport of the proteoglycan to the cell surface of rat liver. *Biochem. J.* **252**: 437–445.

Gupta, D. and Tartakoff, A.M. (1989) Lectin-colloidal gold-induced density perturbation of membranes: application to affinity elimination of the plasma membrane. *Meth. Cell Biol.* **31**: 247–263.

Hashiramoto, M. and James, D.E. (2000) Characterization of Insulin-responsive GLUT4 storage vesicles isolated from 3T3-L1 adipocytes. *Mol. Cell Biol.* **20**: 416–427.

Howell, K.E., Gruenberg, J., Ito, K. and Palade, G. E. (1988) Immunoisolation of subcellular components. In: *Cell Free Analysis of Membrane Traffic* (eds D.J. Morré, K.E. Howell, G.M.C. Cook and W.H. Evans). Alan R Liss Inc., New York, pp. 77–90.

Hubbard, A.L., Wall, D.A. and Ma, A. (1983) Isolation of rat hepatocyte plasma membranes *J. Cell Biol.* **96**: 217–229.

Hubbard, A.L., Dunn, W. A., Mueller, S.C. and Bartles, J.R. (1988) Immunoisolation of hepatocyte membrane compartments using *S. aureus* cell. In: *Cell Free Analysis of Membrane Traffic* (eds D.J. Morré, K.E. Howell, G.M.C. Cook and W.H. Evans). Alan R Liss Inc., New York, pp. 115–127.

Kindberg, G.E., Ford, T., Blomhoff, R., Rickwood, D. and Berg, T. (1984) Separation of endocytic vesicles in Nycodenz gradients. *Anal. Biochem.* **142**: 455–462.

Lafont, F., Verkade, P., Galli, T., Wimmer, C., Louvard, D and Simons, K. (1999) *Proc. Natl.Acad. Sci USA.* **96**: 3734–3738.

Lodish, H.F., Kong, N., Hirani, S. and Rasmussen, J. (1987) A vesicular intermediate in the transport of hepatoma secretory proteins from the rough endoplasmic reticulum to the Golgi complex. *J. Biol. Chem.* **104**: 221–230.

Luzio, J.P. and Richardson, P.J. (1993) Isolation of cholinergic-specific synaptosomes by immunoadsorption. In: *Methods in Molecular Biology*, Vol. 19 (eds J.M. Graham and J.A. Higgins). Humana Press, Totowa, NJ, pp. 141–151.

Macintyre, S.S. (1992) Regulated export of a secretory protein from the ER of the hepatocyte: a specific binding site retaining C-reactive protein within the ER is downregulated during the acute phase response. *J. Cell. Biol.* **118**: 253–265.

Malaba, L., Smeland, S., Senoo, H., Norum, K.R., Berg, T., Blomhoff, R. and Kindberg, G.M. (1995) Retinol-binding protein and asialo-orosomucoid are taken up by different pathways in liver cells. *J. Biol. Chem.* **270**: 15686–15692.

Meier, P.J., Sztul, E.S., Reuben, A. and Boyer, J.L. (1984) Structural and functional polarity of canalicular and basolateral plasma membrane vesicles isolated in high yield from rat liver *J. Cell Biol.* **98**: 991–1000.

Miller, S.G., Carnell, L. and Moore, H.H. (1992) Post-Golgi membrane traffic: brefeldin A inhibits export from distal Golgi compartments to the cell surface but not recycling. *J. Cell Biol.* **118**: 267–283.

Moore, S.E. and Spiro, R.G. (1992) Characterization of the endomannosidase pathway for the processing of N-linked oligosaccharides in glucosidase II-deficient and parent mouse lymphoma cells. *J. Biol. Chem.* **267**: 8443–8451.

Plonné, D., Cartwright, I., Linß, W., Dargel, R., Graham, J.M. and Higgins, J.A. (1999) Separation of the intracellular secretory compartment of rat liver and isolated rat hepatocytes in a single step using self-generated gradients of iodixanol. *Anal. Biochem.* **276**: 88–96.

Scott, L., Schell, M.J. and Hubbard, A.L. (1993) Isolation of plasma membrane sheets and plasma membrane domains from rat liver. In: *Methods in Molecular Biology*, Vol. 19 (eds J.M. Graham and J.A. Higgins). Humana Press, Totowa, NJ, pp. 59–69.

Sheff, D.R., Daro, E.A., Hull, M. and Mellman, I. (1999) The receptor recycling pathway contains two distinct populations of endosomes with different sorting functions. *J. Cell Biol* **145**: 123–139.

Sztul, E.S., Howell, K.E. and Palade, G.E. (1985) Biogenesis of the polymeric IgA receptor in rat hepatocytes II. Localization of its intracellular forms by cell fractionation studies. *J Cell Biol.* **100**: 1255–1261

Tooze, S.A. and Huttner, W.B. (1990) Cell-free sorting to the regulated and constitutive secretory pathways. *Cell* **60**: 837–847.

Uittenbogaard, A., Ying, Y-s. and Smart, E.J (1998) Characterization of a cytosolic heat-shock protein cavelin chaperone complex. *J. Biol Chem.* **273**: 6525–6532.

Yang, M., Ellenberg, J., Bonifacino, J.S. and Weissman, A.M. (1997) The transmembrane domain of a carboxyl-terminal anchored protein determines localization to the endoplasmic reticulum. *J. Biol. Chem.* **272**: 1970–1975.

Zhang, J., Kanh, D.E., Xia, W., Okochi, M., Mori, H., Selkoe, D.J. and Koo, E.H. (1998) Subcellular distribution and turnover of presenilins in transfected cells. *J. Biol. Chem.* **273**: 12436–12442.

Zhou, M., Vallega, G., Kandror, K.V. and Pilch, P.F. (2000) Insulin-mediated translocation of GLUT-4-containing vesicles is preserved in denervated muscles. *Am. J. Physiol Endocrinol. Metab.* **278**: E1019–1026.

Protocol 7.1

Density barrier separation of RER and SER (Bergstrand and Dallner, 1969)

Equipment

High-speed centrifuge with fixed-angle rotor (30–50 ml tubes)

Ultracentrifuge with fixed-angle rotor to accommodate 10–14 ml tubes (e.g. Beckman 50Ti).

Reagents

Homogenization medium (HM): 0.25 M sucrose, 10 mM Tris–HCl, pH 7.4

Sucrose gradient solutions: 1.3 M and 0.6 M sucrose in 15 mM CsCl, 10 mM Tris–HCl, pH 7.4.

Protocol

Carry out all operations at 0–4°C.

1. Prepare a liver homogenate according to *Protocol 6.1* using the above HM.

2. Centrifuge the homogenate at 15 000 g for 20 min.

3. Decant the supernatant.

4. In tubes for the ultracentrifuge rotor layer 3 ml each of the two sucrose solutions.

5. Overlayer the 0.6 M sucrose with the 15 000 g supernatant to fill the tube.

6. Centrifuge at 100 000 g_{av} for 90 min.

7. Remove the interface material (SER).

8. Discard any residual 1.3 M sucrose from above the RER pellet and resuspend the pellet in HM (approximately 10 ml).

9. Dilute the SER fraction with two volumes of HM.

10. Pellet the SER and RER at 100 000 g and resuspend the pellets in an appropriate medium.

Protocol 7.2

Separation of SER and RER on a continuous sucrose gradient (Amar-Costesec *et al.*, 1988)

Equipment

High-speed centrifuge with fixed-angle rotor (30–50 ml tubes)

Ultracentrifuge with fixed-angle rotor for approximately 30 ml tubes (e.g. Beckman 60Ti) and swinging-bucket rotors for approximately 38 ml (e.g. Beckman SW28) or 14 ml tubes (e.g. Beckman SW41)

Two-chamber gradient maker or Gradient Master™

Dounce homogenizer (20–30 ml, loose-fitting).

Reagents

Homogenization medium (HM): 0.25 M sucrose, 10 mM Tris–HCl, pH 7.4

Microsome solution (MS): 0.25 M sucrose, 3 mM imidazole–HCl, pH 8.2

Gradient solutions: 13.6, 17.5, 50, 51.5 and 75% (w/v) sucrose in 3 mM imidazole–HCl, pH 8.2

Stripping solution: 68% (w/v) sucrose, 40 mM pyrophosphate, 3 mM imidazole–HCl, pH 8.2.

Protocol

Carry out all operations at 0–4°C.

1. Prepare a 15 000 g supernatant from a liver homogenate according to *Protocol 7.1* (steps 1–3).

2. Centrifuge at 150 000 g for 30 min in the fixed-angle rotor.

3. Resuspend the pellet in 10–15 ml of MS using the Dounce homogenizer.

4. In tubes for the swinging-bucket rotor prepare a linear gradient using equal volumes of the 17.5 and 51.5% (w/v) sucrose solutions.

5. Underlayer the gradient with the 51.5% cushion and layer the microsomal suspension on top. Use a ratio of sample:gradient:cushion of about 3:2:1.

6. Centrifuge at 100 000 g_{av} for 16 h.

7. The smooth ER bands broadly within the gradient. Harvest this as a single sample (aspirate a volume equal to the sample+gradient) or 1 ml fractions can be aspirated from the meniscus downwards.

8. Resuspend the pellet of rough microsomes in 5 ml of the residual cushion.

9. Adjust the density of this suspension to 1.25 g ml^{-1} (approximately 68% sucrose) by adding 2 volumes of the 75% sucrose solution.

10. Add 5 volumes of stripping solution to 14 vol of suspension.

11. Make a linear 13.6–50% (w/v) linear sucrose gradient in tubes for the swinging-bucket rotor (14-ml tubes); underlay it with the sample (gradient:sample volume ratio of approximatley 3:1) and centrifuge at 200 000 g_{av} in a swinging-bucket rotor for 2 h.

12. The stripped vesicles band broadly between densities 1.10 and 1.19 g ml^{-1}, while peroxisomal (and any mitochondrial) contaminants band below this region.

13. Aspirate the entire band or collect it in a series of 1 ml fractions by upward displacement.

Protocol 7.3

Isolation of Golgi membrane vesicles from an homogenate in a discontinuous sucrose gradient (Balch *et al.*, 1984)

Equipment

Ultracentrifuge with swinging-bucket rotor with approximately 37 ml tubes (e.g. Beckman SW 28).

Reagents

Homogenization medium (HM): 0.25 M sucrose, 10 mM Tris–HCl, pH 7.4

Sucrose gradient solutions: 0.8, 1.2, 1.6 and 2.3 M sucrose in 10 mM Tris–HCl, pH 7.4; for isolating light and heavy fractions: replace the two lower concentrations with 0.86, 1.15 M (Sztul *et al.*, 1985).

Protocol

Carry out all operations at 0–4°C.

For cultured cells: suspend the cells in HM and homogenize using up to 20 strokes of the pestle of the Dounce homogenizer. For liver: prepare a 15 000 g supernatant from a liver homogenate according to *Protocol 7.1* (steps 1–3).

1. Adjust the cell homogenate or 15 000 g supernatant to 1.4 M with respect to sucrose by adding an equal volume of 2.3 M sucrose.

2. Transfer 12 ml to tubes for the swinging-bucket rotor.

3. Overlay the sample with 14 ml of 1.2 M sucrose and 8 ml of 0.8 M sucrose (for light and heavy Golgi fractions overlayer with 14 ml of 1.15 M, 6 ml of 0.86 M and 2 ml of HM).

4. Underlayer the sample with 3 ml of 1.6 M sucrose.

5. Centrifuge at 110 000 g for 2 h.

6. Harvest the Golgi band from the 0.8/1.2 M sucrose interface or the light and dense fractions from the interfaces above and below the 0.86 M sucrose, respectively.

7. If required, harvest the ER which bands within and below the 1.4 M sucrose layer.

Protocol 7.4

Isolation of the hepatocyte sinusoidal membrane domain using immunoaffinity beads (Sztul *et al.*, 1985)

Equipment

Dounce homogenizer (10 ml, loose-fitting)

Shaking water bath at 24°C

High-speed centrifuge with fixed-angle rotor (e.g. Sorvall SS34) and approximately 50 ml tubes

Microcentrifuge with appropriate microcentrifuge tubes

Ultracentrifuge with fixed-angle rotor (e.g. Beckman 50Ti or equivalent) and approximately 13 ml tubes.

Reagents

Anti-SC serum (or other primary antibody)

Nonimmune serum

Protein-Sepharose beads

Solution A: 0.25 M sucrose, 50 mM Tris–HCl, pH 7.4

Solution B: 2% (w/v) Triton X-100, 150 mM NaCl, 2 mM EDTA, 30 mM Tris–HCl, pH, 7.4

Solution C: 1% (w/v) Triton X-100, 0.2% (w/v) SDS, 150 mM NaCl, 5 mM EDTA, 10 mM Tris–HCl, pH 8.0

Medium D: as medium C minus the detergents.

Protocol

Carry out all operations (except where indicated) at 0–4°C.

1. Prepare a 15 000 g supernatant from a 30% (w/v) liver homogenate in solution A according to *Protocol 7.1* (steps 1–3).

2. Centrifuge the supernatant at 120 000 g for 90 min to pellet the microsomes.

3. Resuspend the microsomes (using the Dounce homogenizer) in solution A (at 2 mg microsomal protein ml^{-1}).

4. Incubate 200 μl of a 60% (v/v) suspension of Protein A-Sepharose beads in solution B at 24°C with 50 μl of anti-SC serum (or non-immune serum) for 60 min.

5. Pellet the beads in a microcentrifuge and wash them four times in solution C, and a further two times in the solution D (use a vortex mixer to resuspend the beads in the media).

6. Incubate the beads in 500 µl of the microsome fraction for 2 h at room temperature.

7. Sediment the beads in a microcentrifuge and wash four times in solution A and then finally resuspend in this medium for further analysis.

Protocol 7.5

Analysis of the secretory process in cultured cells using discontinuous sucrose-D$_2$O density gradients (Lodish *et al.*, 1987)

Equipment

Dounce homogenizer (10 ml, tight-fitting)

Gradient unloader (upward displacement)

Low-speed refrigerated centrifuge with swinging-bucket rotor for 10 ml plastic tubes.

Ultracentrifuge with swinging-bucket rotor (e.g. Beckman SW 41Ti).

Reagents

Homogenization buffer (HB): 0.25 M sucrose, 10 mM Hepes–NaOH, pH 7.4

Gradient solutions: 10, 12.5, 15, 17.5, 20, 22.5, 25, 27.5, 30 and 50% (w/v) sucrose, 10 mM Hepes–NaOH, pD 7.4 in D$_2$O.

Protocol

Carry out all operations at 0–4°C.

1. Suspend the cells in HB (use no more than 5 ml).

2. Homogenize using up to 20 strokes of the pestle of the Dounce homogenizer.

3. Pellet the nuclei by centrifugation at 1000 g_{av} for 10 min.

4. Prepare a discontinuous gradient from 1 ml of each of the gradient solutions.

5. Layer 2 ml of the post-nuclear supernatant over the gradient of sucrose and centrifuge at 160 000 g for 3 h in the swinging-bucket rotor.

6. Unload the gradient by upward displacement into approximately 0.3 ml fractions.

Protocol 7.6

Sedimentation velocity gradients (Tooze and Huttner, 1990)

Equipment

Low-speed centrifuge (swinging-bucket rotor for 10–15 ml tubes)

Ultracentrifuge with swinging-bucket rotor (e.g. Beckman SW 41Ti)

Dounce homogenizer (5–10 ml; tight fitting)

Two-chamber gradient maker or Gradient Master™

Gradient unloader (upward displacement).

Reagents

Homogenization medium (HM): 0.25 M sucrose, 1 mM EDTA, 1 mM MgOAc, 10 mM Hepes–KOH, pH 7.2

Sucrose solutions: 0.3, 0.5, 1.2 and 2.0 M in 10 mM Hepes–KOH, pH 7.2.

Protocol

1. Centrifuge the cells at 1700 g_{av} for 5 min

2. Resuspend the pellet in 5–10 times its volume of HM. It is very important to keep the volume of this to a minimum since the first stage of the purification is a sedimentation velocity one.

3. Homogenize the cells using 20 strokes of a tight-fitting Dounce homogenizer and pellet the nuclei and unbroken cells by centrifugation at 1000 g_{av} for 10 min.

4. Prepare a 12.0 ml linear sucrose gradient (0.3–1.2 M) in a tube for the SW41 rotor.

5. Load approx 1.3 ml of supernatant on top.

6. Centrifuge at 78 000 g for 15 min (at speed).

7. Collect 1-ml fractions by upward displacement. The post-TGN vesicles band in the top 4 ml and the TGN in the 8–10 ml region.

8. The collected fractions may be recentrifuged to equilibrium density on any suitable gradient.

Note

As this is a sedimentation velocity separation, if a rotor other than the SW 41Ti is used, it is important that the rotor dimensions should be close to the following: r_{min} = 67 mm; r_{av} = 110 mm; r_{max} = 153 mm.

Protocol 7.7

Fractionation of Golgi, SER and RER in a self-generated iodixanol gradient (Plonné *et al.*, 1999)

Equipment

Dounce homogenizer (loose-fitting, 30 ml)

Gradient unloader (upward displacement)

Ultracentrifuge with vertical or near-vertical rotor (e.g. Beckman VTi65.1) and suitable sealed tubes (approximately 11 ml).

Reagents

Homogenization medium (HM): 0.25 M sucrose, 10 mM Tris–HCl, pH 7.4

OptiPrep™

Diluent: 0.25 M sucrose, 60 mM Tris–HCl, pH 7.4

Working solution (WS) of 50% (w/v) iodixanol: 5 volumes of OptiPrep™ + 1 volume of diluent.

Protocol

Carry out all procedures at 0–4°C.

1. Mince the liver with scissors and then homogenize in HM (4 ml g^{-1} liver) using 30 strokes of the pestle of a loose-fitting Dounce homogenizer.

2. Centrifuge the homogenate at 8000 g for 20 min to pellet most of the larger organelles.

3. Centrifuge the 8000 g supernatant at 100 000 g for 40 min and resuspend the microsomal pellet in HM (5.0 ml per 2 g liver), using 20 strokes of the pestle of the Dounce homogenizer.

4. Mix 2 volumes of the microsome suspension with 3 volumes of working solution.

5. Transfer 4.5 ml to a vertical rotor tube and underlayer with 1.8 ml of 30% (w/v) iodixanol (3 volumes of WS + 2 volumes of HM).

6. Layer approx 4.5 ml of 15% (w/v) iodixanol (1.5 volumes of WS + 3.5 volumes of diluent) on top to fill the tube.

7. Centrifuge at 350 000 g_{av} for 2 h.

8. Collect the gradient in 20 × 0.5 ml fractions by upward displacement with a dense unloading solution.

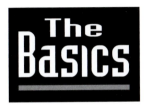

Chapter 8

Fractionation of macromolecules and macromolecular complexes

Except for the use of sucrose gradients to separate proteins and ribonucleo-proteins on the basis of sedimentation rate (Section 2) and the use of KBr gradients for lipoproteins, macromolecules and macromolecular complexes have generally been purified using self-generated gradients of heavy metal salts. Only the iodinated density gradient-media can provide a reasonable substitute to the use of heavy metal salts for fractionating macromolecules and macromolecular complexes. These nonionic iodinated media are ideal for investigating the interactions between macromolecules. New important methods for fractionating viruses (Section 3) and plasma lipoproteins (Section 4) have been established with iodixanol which significantly reduce the centrifugation time. A major attraction of the use of Nycodenz® or iodixanol for macromolecules and macromolecular complexes is that any subsequent analysis of the fractionated products can be carried out without the need to dialyze away the medium.

1. Buoyant density banding of nucleic acids and proteins

1.1 Introduction

Just as the density of osmotically sensitive subcellular particles depends on the movement of water molecules from the gradient medium into the particle, so the density of macromolecules depends on the degree of hydration of the molecule, which in turn is controlled by the availability of free water molecules in the solution. Indeed, the effect of the water activity of the gradient medium can have an even more startling effect on the density of a macromolecule than the effect of osmolality on the density of a subcellular particle. Those solutions, which contain a large number of free water molecules, are said to possess a high water activity and such a solution would also have a low osmolality (although the two functions are not truly reciprocal). At the concentration range of CsCl gradients used to band nucleic acids isopycnically (3–6 M), most of the water molecules are associated with the solute particles, so that the number of water molecules available for association with each nucleotide residue is less than eight, on the other hand in Nycodenz® gradients that number is 50 or more (Ford and Rickwood, 1983). Consequently, the density of nucleic acids in CsCl is much greater than in Nycodenz®. The density of DNA in iodixanol is even lower than in

Nycodenz®, being approximately 1.11 gml⁻¹. Another consequence of the low water activity of CsCl solutions is that density of RNA is so high that this nucleic acid cannot be banded in CsCl gradients (it will always pellet) and can only be banded in $CsSO_4$ gradients in which it has a lower density (*Table 8.1*).

The amount of water that associates with proteins, even in solutions of high water activity (Nycodenz® and iodixanol) is relatively low, so their density in CsCl (approximately 1.33 gml⁻¹) is only slightly higher than that in either of the two iodinated density gradient media (1.26 g ml⁻¹). *Table 8.1* gives the density of a number of macromolecules in a small selection of gradient media; this is described more fully in Rickwood (1992). Because the density of all proteins in a particular gradient medium is approximately the same, irrespective of molecular mass, different proteins can usually only be separated on the basis of their sedimentation velocity (see Section 2), although because polysaccharides have a slightly higher density, particularly in CsCl (the difference is rather less than in iodinated density gradient media), it may be possible to fractionate highly glycosylated proteins and proteoglycans. The steepness of CsCl gradients however makes them not well suited for the fractionation of proteins. Fractionation of proteins and glycoproteins are rather more effective in RbCl gradients.

1.2   Self-generated gradients for fractionation of nucleic acids

For many years, self-generated gradients of heavy metals salts and of CsCl in particular were used as the standard media for the fractionation of nucleic acids. Some of the classic studies on DNA replication were carried out in self-generated CsCl or $CsSO_4$ gradients. CsCl gradients can efficiently separate supercoiled, linear and relaxed-circular DNA and they are especially useful for the preparation of purified plasmid DNA (see Section 1.4).

Separation of DNA species with different base composition

G–C base pairs are less highly hydrated than A–T base pairs and hence a DNA molecule with a high G–C content will have a higher density than one with a high A–T content and the banding density of the DNA in the gradient can be used to calculate the G+C content (Rickwood and Chambers, 1984).

Table 8.1. Buoyant density (g/ml⁻¹) of macromolecules in density gradient media

Macromolecule	CsCl	Cs₂SO₄	Metrizamide	Nycodenz®	Iodixanol
Native DNA	1.71	1.43	1.12	1.13	1.12
Denatured DNA	1.73	1.45	1.14	1.17	1.16
RNA	>1.9	1.64	1.17	1.18	1.18
Polysaccharides	1.62		1.28	1.29	
Proteins	1.3	1.3	1.27	1.27	1.26
Proteoglycans		1.46			

Data from Ford and Rickwood (1983), Rickwood (1992) and Rickwood and Patel (1996).

Nucleic acid synthesis

Pulse-chase radiolabeling with a heavy isotope such as ^{15}N or incorporation of a dense nucleotide analog (e.g. bromodeoxyuridine) can be used to study the synthesis of DNA and RNA. The density shift caused by the incorporation of ^{15}N is 0.016 g ml^{-1}, while the analog can shift the density by 0.08 g ml^{-1} (Rickwood and Chambers, 1984).

Separation of DNA/RNA hybrids from DNA and RNA

Because RNA is so much denser than DNA (in any gradient medium), self-generated gradients are very effective for studying separating the free macro-molecules and also hybrids of the two molecules (see *Figure 8.1*). In Cs_2SO_4 RNA has a lower buoyant density and therefore this medium may be used not only for the isopycnic banding of DNA, DNA/RNA hybrids and protein, but for RNA as well, but the downside of this is that the steepness of the gradient does not permit such good separation of native and denatured DNA. One problem which might arise with Cs_2SO_4 is that high-molecular-weight RNA may aggregate and precipitate in the presence of sulfate ions (Rickwood and Chambers, 1984).

   The centrifugation conditions which are chosen must be sufficient to band the macromolecules according to their buoyant density on the one hand and on the other create and maintain an appropriate gradient-density profile to achieve the required resolution. A commonly used strategy is to use a very high relative centrifugal field (RCF) to permit the rapid banding

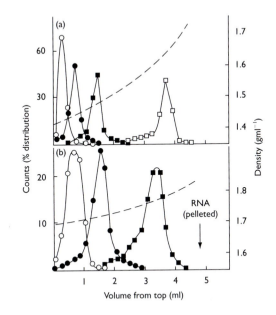

Figure 8.1

Fractionation of nucleic acids in gradients of heavy metal salts. Native DNA (○), denatured DNA (●), RNA (□) and DNA-RNA hybrids (■) were banded by isopycnic centrifugation in self-generated gradients of (a) CsSO$_4$ (1.54 g ml^{-1} starting density) or (b) CsCl (1.75 g ml^{-1} starting density). For more information see text. Adapted from Rickwood (1992) Preparative Centrifugation – A Practical Approach *with kind permission of the author and IRL Press at Oxford University Press.*

of the macromolecules in a steep gradient and then to reduce the speed to allow the formation of a shallow gradient in the middle of the tube for achieving high resolution. This process is known as gradient relaxation. Some of the parameters controlling the formation of self-generated gradients are covered in Chapter 4 but for a more complete discussion of the theory behind choice of the correct gradient forming conditions for DNA banding, see Rickwood and Chambers (1984). Choice of the correct rotor and centrifugation conditions is particularly important for CsCl gradients, since too high an RCF for too long a time can create such a high density at the bottom of the gradient that the maximum density permitted for the rotor may be exceeded. In fixed-angle and swinging-bucket rotors in particular, in which this very high density is created in a small volume at the bottom of the tube, the stress is concentrated over a small area of the rotor tube pocket and may lead to rotor failure. In near-vertical and vertical rotors the stress is less marked since the dense layer is distributed over the full length of the tube.

1.3   Interactions between nucleic acid and proteins

There are two types of interactions between nucleic acids and proteins that are important in the control and regulation of transcription and translation – ionic and sequence-specific. These interactions may be relatively unstable and they are certainly influenced by the ionic environment of the molecules. Thus the use of highly ionic CsCl gradients does not permit the study of such interactions. Gradients of iodinated density-gradient media on the other hand, which are nonionic, are unlikely to interfere with these processes and it is possible to investigate modulation of the ionic environment on these events. Ford and Rickwood (1983) have made a number of studies on the binding of histone and nonhistone proteins to DNA.

While macromolecular complexes such as ribonucleoprotein particles can be isolated in CsCl gradients, it is certainly more valid to investigate the binding between proteins and RNA in nonionic gradients rather than ionic ones. This is especially the case when the effect of the binding of various ions on these interactions and on the buoyant density of macromolecules is being studied Ford and Rickwood (1983). Clearly, the normal ionic media (solutions of heavy metal salts) cannot be used for such studies.

1.4   Separation of plasmid DNA

Perhaps one of the most important modern uses of density gradients is the purification of plasmid DNA. Native DNAs of the same base composition and molecular mass but of different conformation band at the same density in CsCl gradients. The only way of separating the native molecules is therefore on the basis of sedimentation velocity (rate-zonal). Another more convenient approach is to use an intercalating agent such as ethidium bromide (EtBr). Intercalation of EtBr between the bases of DNA reduces the density of the molecule and the amount of EtBr that intercalates depends on the conformation of the DNA. Superhelical DNA binds less EtBr than linear DNA and in this manner the density of linear DNA is decreased by 0.19 g ml^{-1} while that of plasmid DNA is decreased by only 0.13 g ml^{-1} (in the presence of saturation amounts of the intercalating agent). Intercalation of the EtBr also provides a useful means of identifying the positions of the plasmid and chromosomal

DNA in the gradient as they can be visualized under UV light by a red fluorescence. This methodology is described in *Protocol 8.1*. For a more detailed treatment of this topic, see Rickwood (1992).

This technique became very popular in the 1970s and 1980s, however, it suffers from a number of problems. The corrosive nature of CsCl, the necessity to remove CsCl by dialysis prior to agarose-gel electrophoresis, its precipitation by ethanol, its cost and its general incompatibility to biological material have all contributed to the lack of popularity of centrifugation for DNA preparation. In addition, as discussed above, the density of CsCl gradients at the r_{max} may be close to the maximum permissible value for some rotors; this may overstress the rotor and potentially be catastrophic (although the use of vertical and near-vertical rotors alleviates this problem). The other significant drawback is the hazardous nature of EtBr; as it intercalates DNA it is thus a potent mutagen. For these reasons, when alternative column chromatographic techniques became available, the popularity of the method declined, even though density gradient centrifugation probably achieves the best purification of plasmid DNA of any method.

In an alternative technique, iodixanol replaces CsCl and the blue-fluorescent marker 4,6-diamidino-2-phenylindole (DAPI) replaces EtBr. It has several advantages over the CsCl–EtBr method. As iodixanol is nonionic plasmid DNA can be analyzed by electrophoresis directly without dialysis; iodixanol is not precipitated by propan-2-ol or ethanol, nor does it inhibit restriction nucleases. Densities of nucleic acids in iodixanol (approximately $1.10 \, \mathrm{g \, ml^{-1}}$) are much lower than in CsCl: the gradients required are thus of a much lower density and cannot stress rotors. Also because DAPI binds in the groove of the DNA it is very much less hazardous than EtBr. In this method (*Protocol 8.2*) the plasmid DNA is less dense than the chromosomal DNA (Rickwood and Patel, 1996). *Figure 8.2* compares the separation of plasmid DNA, chromosomal DNA and RNA in CsCl–EtBr and iodixanol-DAPI gradients.

2. Rate-zonal (sedimentation-velocity) banding of proteins and ribonucleoproteins

Rate-zonal centrifugation is used principally in two areas: the fractionation of proteins of different molecular mass and of a range of ribonucleoprotein particles such as ribosomal subunits, ribosomes and polysomes.

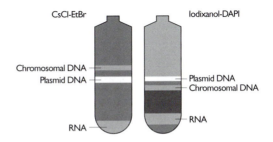

Figure 8.2

Banding of plasmid DNA in CsCl–ethidium bromide (EtBr) and iodixanol–4,6-diamidino-2-phinylindole (DAPI) gradients. Chrom-DNA, chromosomal DNA. See Protocols 8.1 and 8.2 for experimental details.

2.1 Proteins

Broadly speaking, all proteins have a similar density (in any gradient medium) irrespective of their molecular mass (although there are some minor differences in density which reflect the variable hydration of different amino acids). Thus fractionation of proteins according to molecular mass is carried out by sedimentation velocity in rate-zonal gradients. These techniques can also provide information on protein–protein interactions and may even detect large changes in conformation due to ligand binding. This short section only considers the use of standard centrifugation hardware for analyzing proteins; analytical centrifugation, which can provide much more, detailed information about molecular mass, shape, hydrodynamic radius, conformation, dimensions and interactions with other molecules, is beyond the scope of this basic text. A short description of the technique is given in Chapter 1 (Section 11) but for more information about its uses for analyzing macromolecules, see Eason (1984). Although the use of the various types of polyacrylamide gel electrophoresis (PAGE) and isoelectric focusing (combined with electroblotting) has largely superceded the use of density-gradient centrifugation for the determination of molecular mass and fractionation of proteins, there are certain types of protein which behave anomalously in such systems. In sodium dodecyl sulfate (SDS)–PAGE glycoproteins, proteoglycans and highly charged proteins bind the detergent atypically making their behavior in these systems erratic and the data on their molecular mass unreliable.

Choice of gradient

The most common choice of gradient for protein analysis is sucrose and a 5–20% (w/w) sucrose gradient is a good starting point for any protein fractionation experiment and will give good resolution in most swinging-bucket or vertical rotors. This gradient is essentially isokinetic, that is, the retarding forces experienced by the protein molecules as they move down gradient due to the increase in density and viscosity of the medium are almost exactly counterbalanced by the acceleration forces due to the increase in RCF. Thus the molecules move through the gradient at an approximately constant rate – an ideal situation for resolving particles according to size. Sucrose is also a popular choice for these sedimentation-velocity gradients since it does not interact with the majority of proteins (see *Protocol 8.3*). If sucrose does appear to interfere with protein sedimentation then a glycerol gradient covering the same concentration range provides an alternative that behaves almost identically to sucrose.

More recently OptiPrep™ has been introduced for the fractionation of proteins by Basi and Rebois (1997). The strategy takes advantage of the ability of iodixanol to form self-generated gradients. Particularly when comparisons are being made between the sedimentation velocity of a protein in the presence and absence of a some modifying agent, it is necessary to assure that each gradient-density profile is identical. It is therefore important that the conditions for preparing a pre-formed gradient of sucrose or glycerol are precisely controlled. This can sometimes be difficult and tedious. By forming the gradient from identical volumes of a uniform concentration of iodixanol using the centrifugal field, the identity of gradients in each tube is assured.

The method does, however, require a rotor with a short sedimentation path-length. On the other hand this also means that the method works optimally with relatively small volumes of gradient and sample – often important when amounts of material may be limited (*Protocol 8.4*).

It will also be necessary to include in the gradient (in addition to a suitable buffer) a variety of additives (which will also be in the sample); commonly these might be EDTA, dithiothreitol, divalent cations and a suitable detergent. In other instances it might be necessary to include urea or guanidinium chloride in order to keep the protein in a soluble form to prevent adventitious aggregation with other protein molecules and to keep it functionally intact.

Choice of rotor and centrifugation conditions

A commonly used rotor for these rate zonal sucrose gradients is a swinging-bucket rotor with 5-ml tubes capable of approximately 300 000 g_{max}, for example, the Beckman SW50.1 or Sorvall AH650. Centrifugation normally is carried out for approximately 16 h. The actual centrifugation conditions will have to be carried out by trial and error unless the sedimentation coefficients of the molecules are known. In which case, there are a number of computer programs which will define the centrifugation conditions for a particular rotor type and gradient-density profile (see Young, 1984; Steensgard *et al.*, 1992, for more details).

As with all rate-zonal separations the volume of sample must be kept as small as possible so that the protein molecules move through the gradient as narrow zones. The use of swinging-bucket rotors, which have relatively long sedimentation path-lengths, are potentially ideal for achieving good separation between proteins of different molecular mass. However, the downside of this is the relatively long centrifugation time during which the protein may lose activity. Another time-dependent problem is diffusion, which will lead to band broadening. This is not a serious problem with the large particles that we have been considering in earlier chapters but for particles <200 kDa, diffusion becomes significant and the smaller the protein the greater will be the rate of diffusion.

Therefore it might be considered that the use of a near-vertical or vertical rotor might be of great benefit for such separations. Not only is the sample zone very narrow but also the short sedimentation path-length will mean correspondingly shorter centrifugation times (see Chapter 2). However, because of the wide surface area of the gradient and the short distance between the top and bottom of the gradient, the effect of diffusion may cause even more serious band broadening. Fixed-angle rotors might provide a useful compromise and so long as there are no serious wall effects (i.e. the protein molecules do not adhere to the tube wall) then these can be effectively used. Indeed, a small-volume fixed-angle rotor was used by Basi and Rebois (1997) in their experiments and it provided resolution which was comparable with a routine swinging-bucket rotor (see below) and the fractionation took only 1 h.

Irrespective of the chosen rotor type, but particularly for fixed-angle, near-vertical and vertical rotors in which the sample zone and gradient reorient in the tube, slow acceleration to and deceleration from 2000 r.p.m. is essential to maintain the highest resolution.

The sedimentation coefficients ($s_{20,w}$) of a series of proteins of different molecular mass are given in *Table 8.2* and in *Figure 8.3* the rate-zonal banding of a selection of these proteins is shown in a 5-ml 5–20% (w/v) sucrose gradient centrifuged at 43 000 r.p.m. for 17 h in a Beckman SW 50.1. For comparison, a sucrose gradient of the same density range (0.2 ml in volume) was run in a Beckman TLA120.2 for 1 h at 120 000 r.p.m. In the case of OptiPrep™, 0.2 ml of a 30% (w/v) iodixanol was centrifuged at 100 000 r.p.m. in the TLA120.2 for 3 h to generate the linear gradient and then after deceleration to zero the protein solution was layered on top of the gradient and recentrifuged at 120 000 r.p.m. for 1 h. When the peak distances migrated by each protein are plotted against the $s_{20,w}$ a linear relationship is produced in all three situations.

Table 8.2. Sedimentation coefficients of proteins of different molecular mass

Protein	Molecular mass	$s_{20,w}$
α-Lactalbumin	14 200	1.92
Lysozyme	14 300	2.19
Soyabean trypsin inhibitor	20 100	2.30
Carbonic anhydrase	29 000	2.80
Ovalbumin	45 000	3.54
Bovine serum albumin	66 000	4.41
Transferrin	81 000	4.90

Data partly from Basi and Rebois (1997).

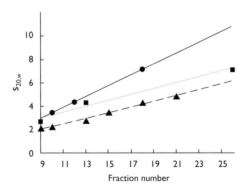

Figure 8.3

*Analysis of proteins by sedimentation velocity in sucrose and iodixanol gradients. Soluble proteins were analyzed on a self-generated iodixanol (30% starting concentration) gradient (■) or a pre-formed (5–20%) sucrose gradient (▲), in a 200-μl tube for a fixed-angle rotor at 250 000g for 1–2 h or a pre-formed sucrose gradient in a 5-ml tube for a swinging bucket rotor (●) at 220 000g for 17 h. For experimental details see Protocols 8.3 and 8.4. The peak protein position (fraction number) is plotted as a function of its sedimentation coefficient ($S_{20,w}$). Adapted from Basi and Rebois (1997) Anal. Biochem. **251**: 103–109, with kind permission of the authors and Academic Press.*

Gradient collection

To be able to analyze proteins in these gradients in a reproducible and accurate fashion it is necessary to use a gradient unloading device which maintains high resolution. The two devices described in Chapter 4 which aspirate the gradient from the top with a probe which is advanced down through the gradient by a motor are the best suited to this requirement. Alternatively, tube puncture and collection dense end first, or the use of upward displacement using a dense medium delivered by tube puncture can be used. However, for the small-volume gradients it is necessary to use one of the aspiration from the top devices.

Practical note

If iodixanol is used, note that 280 nm absorbance cannot be used to monitor the protein distribution because the gradient medium interferes in the ultraviolet (UV).

2.2 Ribonucleoproteins

Although there are some significant differences in the banding density of ribonucleoprotein particles in CsCl gradients, because of the high ionic strength of CsCl solutions, the nucleoproteins need to be fixed prior to centrifugation, which makes the technique of little use. In sucrose, different ribonucleoprotein particles tend to have overlapping densities but rate-zonal (sedimentation-velocity) separations can be very effective for the fractionation of these particles. Generally, low RCFs are used for these gradients to avoid disruption of the delicate structures of ribonucleoproteins.

It is beyond the scope of this text to present a comprehensive description of all of the modern uses of rate-zonal density gradients to analyze ribosomes and polysomes. However, a system that is often used as a source of polysomes is given in *Protocol 8.5*. In exponentially growing *Escherichia coli* most of the ribosomes are engaged in protein synthesis and rate-zonal sucrose gradients can be used to separate the more rapidly sedimenting polysomes from run-off ribosomes (70S) and the smaller slowly sedimenting ribosomal subunits (*Figure 8.4*). The polysomes fractionate into tetra-, tri- and disomes and the subunits from prokaryotic systems are characterized by their sedimentation coefficient (50S and 30S). Efficient preparation of polysomes requires the use of low temperature (preferably <4°C) and a rapid a preparation time as possible.

Rat liver is also a common source of both ribosomes and ribosomal subunits. The post-mitochondrial supernatant is a rich source of rough endoplasmic reticulum from which ribosomes can be released by treatment with deoxycholate and dissociated by puromycin. Ribosomes can be subsequently purified by sedimentation through a 1 M sucrose cushion and after dissociation the 40S and 60S subunits are separated on a 15–30% (w/v) sucrose gradient at 30 000 *g* for 14 h (*Protocol 8.6*).

A more thorough description of methods for the functional analysis of protein translation can be found in Bommer *et al.* (1997). In Nycodenz® there are some significant differences in the densities of certain ribonucleoprotein particles but the actual densities depend both on the cell or tissue type and the ionic composition of the gradient, see Houssais (1983) for more information.

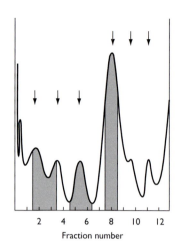

Figure 8.4

Sedimentation velocity separation of E. coli *ribosomal particles in a 10–40% sucrose gradient. The three arrows on the left indicate the position of tetra-, tri- and disomes (left to right); the three arrows on the right (top) indicate the position of run-off 70-S ribosomes, 50-S and 30-S subunits (left to right). The gradient was collected dense-end first, for experimental details see* Protocol 8.5. *Adapted from Bommer* et al. *(1997) in Subcellular Fractionation – A Practical Approach (eds. J.M. Graham and D. Rickwood), IRL Press at Oxford University Press. With kind permission of Oxford University Press.*

3.   Viruses

3.1   Introduction

The concentration and purification of viruses from culture fluid is an important prerequisite not only for studying the structure and function of the particles themselves, but also as part of any ongoing program of virus culture and as a preliminary procedure for the production of vaccines. Some of the important animal RNA viruses have quite different sizes and densities: poliovirus and Coxsackie virus, for example, are both relatively small (20–30 nm; sedimentation coefficient approximately 150S); they are spherical naked nucleocapsids containing RNA and a small number of polypeptides. Semliki Forest virus is rather larger (40–70 nm; sedimentation coefficient approximately 280S) and is surrounded by a host cell-derived envelope, while the measles virus which is also enveloped is even larger (>150 nm; sedimentation coefficient >1000S). There are numerous problems in isolating any virus, even with the simpler naked nucleocapsid types, there are viral precursors of a range of sizes and the enveloped viruses have banding densities not unlike some of the denser membranous organelles of the cells in which they were growing.

The technology of virus purification by centrifugation was principally worked out in the 1960s and because of the frequent requirement to process large volumes of virus-containing fluid, a lot of the protocols were elaborated using either batch-type or continuous-flow zonal rotors (Chapter 2). These methods can, however, be adapted to a smaller scale using routine vertical, fixed-angle and swinging-bucket rotors. Centrifugation strategies for purifying viruses have remained more or less unchanged until the last 4–5 years, when the use of viral vectors to introduce genetic material into cells, as part of a potential gene therapy scheme, became an area of intensive research. Although density-gradient centrifugation has been retained as part of the overall viral purification processing, it often has to be compatible with subsequent preparative (principally chromatographic) and analytical methods.

3.2 Gradient media, virus density and infectivity

See Vanden Berghe (1983) for a comprehensive review of the effect of gradient media on viruses.

Inorganic salts

Particularly because of the nucleic acid and protein composition of non-enveloped viruses (such as poliovirus and Coxsackie virus) and their consequently relatively high density, CsCl has been a popular medium for the density banding of viruses; in this medium some viruses have a density of at least 1.3 g ml^{-1} (*Table 8.3*). Enveloped viruses such as measles virus and Semliki Forest virus display somewhat lower densities, presumably because of the lipid content of their surrounding membranes. Indeed, the lower density of enveloped viruses is generally observed with all gradient media. Although inorganic salts can provide the requisite high density, they tend to be rather toxic and there is evidence that exposure of any virus to such media causes a variable loss of infectivity (*Table 8.4*). Generally, however, the nonenveloped viruses are relatively insensitive and show rather little loss of infectivity.

Table 8.3. Buoyant density (g ml^{-1}) of viruses in different gradient media

Virus type	CsCl	Sucrose	Nycodenz®	Iodixanol
Poliovirus	1.34	1.18–1.26	1.30–1.31	1.19–1.21
Semliki Forest virus	1.26	1.18	1.18	
Measles virus	1.21	1.18	1.18	
Retrovirus				1.17–1.19
Herpes virus	1.27	1.22		1.16–1.18

Data partly taken from Vanden Berghe (1983).

Table 8.4. Effect of gradient medium on recovery of virus infectivity (% of control)

Virus type	CsCl	Sucrose	Nycodenz®	Iodixanol
Poliovirus	40	100	100	100
Measles virus	16	50	16	
Semliki Forest virus	20	77	77	
Astrovirus				100
Herpes virus	40–50			100
Recombinant AAV	1–60			26–100

Data partly taken from Vanden Berghe (1983) and Hermens *et al.* (1999).
AAV, adeno-associated virus.

Sucrose

Compared to CsCl, sucrose is notably less toxic to most viruses and has almost no effect whatsoever on the nonenveloped viruses (*Table 8.4*). Densities are also notably lower in sucrose than in inorganic salts. The reason for this is not entirely clear, it may be related to the lower osmolality of sucrose gradients; however, in gradients of much lower osmolality (see below) the density of viruses may not be significantly lower than in sucrose.

Iodinated density-gradient media

Because of the generally more 'particle-friendly' nature of these gradient media (compared to both CsCl and sucrose), these media tend to promote the retention of good viral infectivity (*Table 8.4*), although it is clear that there may be important differences in the response of particular viruses. Measles virus, for instance, is apparently very sensitive to metrizamide; this may be related to the presence of a glucosamine residue in this molecule (metrizamide is also toxic to certain mammalian cells). Therefore it is wise to check on the effect of a density-gradient medium on viral infectivity before using a particular separation protocol. It has now been shown that in iodixanol a number of viruses, including retrovirus (Møller-Larsen and Christensen, 1998), human immunodeficiency virus (Dettenhoffer and Yu, 1999) and recombinant adeno-associated virus (Hermens *et al.*, 1999; Zolotukhin *et al.*, 1999), retain considerably greater infectivity than in comparable CsCl or sucrose gradients.

The density of both enveloped and nonenveloped viruses in these iodinated density-gradient media is certainly considerably lower than in CsCl and either similar to or slightly lower than in sucrose (*Table 8.3*). However, again there are some virus-type-specific exceptions; poliovirus, for example, is apparently denser in Nycodenz® than it is in sucrose. The apparent density of viruses may also be affected by the composition of the buffer used in the gradient, most notably the presence of either divalent cations or a chelating agent. In iodixanol the densities of viruses cover a slightly lower density range as Nycodenz® ($1.16–1.22$ g ml^{-1}), although the two media have not been compared directly with the same viruses. Recombinant adeno-associated virus (rAAV) has a slightly higher density in iodixanol than other viruses ($1.24–1.26$ g ml^{-1}).

Plant viruses, at least in Nycodenz®, tend to be rather denser than their animal counterparts, banding generally in the range $1.24–1.27$ g ml^{-1} (Gugerli, 1984).

3.3 Purification strategies

The processing of virus is accomplished in four or five stages:

1. Release of the viral particles from the host cells or from other growth environments such as the allantoic fluid of eggs.
2. Clarification of the virus containing fluid by low speed centrifugation at $1000–2000$ *g* for 20–30 min at $4\,^{\circ}$C to remove nuclei, debris and unbroken cells.
3. Concentration of the virus.
4. Purification of the virus from other cellular contaminants.
5. Removal of the density gradient medium (optional).

Release of viral particles

Release from cells may be carried out either by gentle sonication or treatment of the cells with a nonionic detergent such as Triton X-100 or Nonidet NP40. In the case of allantoic fluid, this stage merely requires aspiration of the fluid through a puncture hole made in the shell.

Concentration of virus

This procedure maybe carried out by high-speed or ultracentrifugation of the clarified fluid in order to pellet the virus. The actual RCF required will depend on the size of the virus; some of the larger viruses may be sedimented at approximately 50 000 g for 1–2 h (i.e. it is possible to use a fixed-angle rotor in a high-speed centrifuge). For some of the smaller viruses it is more convenient to use an ultracentrifuge and RCFs of 100 000–200 000 g for 30 min are commonly used. One of the problems of this approach is that other cellular organelles will also be sedimented along with the virus and serious aggregation can occur, so that it may even be necessary to use mild sonication to disperse the pellet in the suspension medium. An unfortunate side-effect of these pelleting and dispersal processes is that loss of viral infectivity is often observed at this stage. This can be avoided by banding the virus on to a cushion of dense medium.

Purification

Purification is normally achieved by equilibrium density banding. Because of the variety of virus sizes and densities, it is normally necessary to customize the gradient and centrifugation conditions to each specific virus. The aim, however, of this step is to achieve removal of membranes and organelles from the host cell. While most of these are likely to be less dense than the virus particles, it is possible that peroxisomes and some ribonucleoprotein particles may co-purify with the virus. This step is also likely to achieve some further concentration.

Recently, however, a number of separations have been based on a rate-zonal method in a continuous iodixanol gradient, first devised for human immunodeficiency virus by Dettenhoffer and Yu (1999).

Protocol 8.7 describes the isolation of Sendai virus (an enveloped virus) using a two-stage process: a sucrose barrier to concentrate the virus, followed by a discontinuous sucrose gradient to purify the virus.

Protocol 8.8 describes a single discontinuous gradient of iodixanol for the purification of rAAV from 30–40 ml of clarified virus-containing fluid. The gradient is able to separate rAAV from adenovirus, contaminating membranes and soluble proteins (Zolotukhin *et al.*, 1999).

Iodixanol permits the purification of a virus in a self-generated gradient and a very effective method is to concentrate the virus on to a dense cushion of 50% iodixanol (compare the sucrose barrier technique of *Protocol 8.7*), followed by banding in a self-generated gradient (see the flowchart in *Figure 8.5* and *Protocol 8.9*). The banding of Herpes virus in this self-generated system displays a sharp band of infectivity at a density of approximately 1.17 g ml^{-1} (*Figure 8.6*).

Often the infectivity profile within a gradient does not display a single well-defined peak; a significant spread of infectivity in the gradient is observed. The most commonly observed pattern is a major dense peak with

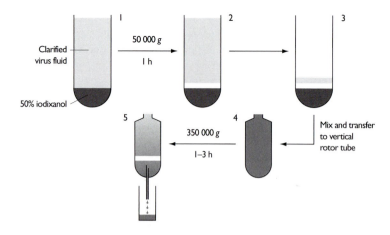

Figure 8.5

Strategy for purifying virus using a self-generated gradient of iodixanol. In step 3, all of the supernatant is removed except for a volume equivalent to that of the 50% (w/v) iodixanol cushion so that in the tube for the vertical rotor, the iodixanol concentration is 25%.

lower levels of infectivity being detected broadly at lower densities or sometimes there is a defined minor low-density peak (*Figure 8.6*). This can be observed in a variety of media. In a few cases the reverse may also be observed, that is, the low-density material forms the major band in the gradient. This broad spread of infectivity is not surprising as the total virus particle population will include both mature and immature forms, some of which may be lacking in certain coat proteins or (in the case of enveloped viruses) lacking the limiting membrane.

 Removal of the gradient medium may or may not be necessary, depending on the type of gradient medium that is used and the nature of the subsequent

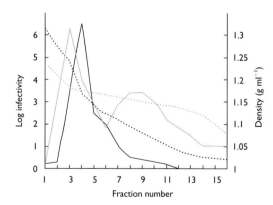

Figure 8.6

Purification of Herpes virus in self-generated iodixanol gradients. The method used is described in Figure 8.5 and Protocol 8.9. Infectivity (solid lines) and density (dotted lines) profiles are compared after centrifugation in the vertical rotor for 2.5 h (black) or 1 h (gray). By changing the shape of the density profile the low-density shoulder observed on the low-density side of the major peak at 2.5 h is resolved as a discrete lower-density population of viral particles after 1 h (see Protocol 8.9).

virus processing. This may be performed by dialysis, by centrifugal ultrafiltration or by dilution of the gradient material with buffer (to reduce its density and viscosity) followed by recovery of the virus by sedimentation. Choice of procedure can be critical because of the potential loss of infectivity that can occur due either to pelleting of the virus or the extra time (normally 12–16 h) required for dialysis. Ultrafiltration through filters (with a 100-kDa cut-off) that fit into tubes for a standard microcentrifuge is normally only practical on relatively small volumes of sample, but it is very rapid.

4. Plasma lipoproteins

4.1 Introduction

Although there are a number of techniques for fractionating plasma lipoproteins (e.g. electrophoresis), density-gradient centrifugation has always been the 'gold-standard' method and it is the only method which can be used preparatively. Indeed, lipoproteins are principally categorized on the basis of their density: high-density (HDL), low-density (LDL) and very low-density (VLDL); chylomicrons have the lowest density of all. HDL, LDL and VLDL are each characterized by a particular range of banding densities as measured in density gradients of potassium bromide (*Table 8.5*). The density differences are caused primarily by different lipid:protein ratios, thus the lipid:protein ratio (and size) increases from HDL to VLDL. Chylomicrons have the highest lipid:protein ratio and size by far, and because their density is so low (<0.99 g ml^{-1}) they are routinely removed from the plasma by flotation prior to fractionation of the other lipoproteins in a density gradient.

Since HDL, LDL and VLDL are operationally identified by their density ranges, it is clear that each lipoprotein class is heterogeneous and comprises a spectrum of particles of different densities and sizes. Recently it has become apparent that the risk of coronary artery disease is particularly linked with the prevalence of small high-density LDL particles, which appear to be intimately involved with the uptake of cholesterol into the cells lining the artery walls. This has provided a catalyst for renewed interest in lipoprotein fractionation techniques.

4.2 Fractionation in KBr by sequential flotation

Raising the density of a suspension of particles, so that the density is just greater than the least dense particle so that only this particle will float to the top of the liquid during centrifugation, is a commonly used and simple

Table 8.5. Density (g ml^{-1}) of human plasma lipoproteins in KBr and iodixanol

Lipoprotein	KBr	Iodixanol
VLDL	<1.006	<1.006
LDL	1.019–1.063	1.010–1.030
HDL	1.063–1.210	1.030–1.140

Data from Graham *et al.* (1996)
VLDL, very low-density lipoprotein; LDL, low-density lipoprotein; HDL, high-density lipoprotein.

procedure (see Chapter 4). In sequential flotation the density of the remaining medium is raised stepwise so that subsequent centrifugations allow the recovery, by flotation, of particles of increasing density. This incremental increase in density is achieved by direct dissolution of solid KBr in each infrantant (Mackness and Durrington, 1992). This time-consuming procedure (flotation of the three major classes of lipoprotein requires three overnight centrifugations) is widely used because the alternative technique of using discontinuous and continuous gradients of such a low-viscosity medium is technically difficult (see Section 4.3).

The density of plasma is approximately 1.03 g ml^{-1}, but during centrifugation the plasma proteins will sediment and the density of the bulk of the liquid above the proteins (the small solute density) will reduce to approximately 1.006 g ml^{-1} (the same as normal saline). Thus during the centrifugation of chylomicron-free plasma only the VLDL ($<$1.006 g ml^{-1}) will be of sufficiently low density to float to the surface. After removal of the VLDL, KBr is added to the remaining plasma so that during the next centrifugation the 'small solute' density of the plasma increases to approximately 1.063 g ml^{-1} and the LDL will float to the surface. Finally, after removal of the LDL more KBr is dissolved in the residual plasma to allow the HDL (density $<$1.21 g ml^{-1}) to float to the surface during the final centrifugation. Sequential flotation is normally carried out in a fixed-angle rotor and it is described in *Protocol 8.10*.

Practical note

The procedure illustrates a potentially important problem in the balancing of centrifuge rotors. During centrifugation of the plasma, the density profile of the liquid in the tube changes dramatically. In the first step to isolate the VLDL for example, initially the density is uniform and approximately 1.03 g ml^{-1} (the density of 0.25 M sucrose). During centrifugation, however, the density profile of the liquid will progressively change as the proteins sediment and the VLDL floats to the surface. By the end of the centrifugation the bulk of the liquid phase will be devoid of proteins (ρ = 1.006 g ml^{-1}) but the density will increase exponentially towards the bottom of the tube to approximately 1.3 g ml^{-1}. Hence it is not satisfactory to balance a tube containing plasma with one containing 0.15 M NaCl (ρ = 1.006 g ml^{-1}) or 0.25 M sucrose (ρ = 1.03 g ml^{-1}), since in both these solutions the density will be remain uniform throughout the centrifugation. In such cases all tubes should contain the plasma.

4.3   Fractionation in KBr gradients

An interesting approach to the problem of separating plasma lipoproteins in a continuous gradient of KBr was devised by Chung *et al.* (1986). The plasma is adjusted to a high density (e.g. 1.30 g ml^{-1}) and layered under a KBr solution of low density (e.g. 1.006 g ml^{-1}) in a tube for a vertical rotor. Because the reorientation of the layers during acceleration creates layers of a large surface area and a small linear thickness, diffusion rapidly creates a linear gradient in which the lipoproteins band according to their density.

4.4   Self-generated iodixanol gradients

Sequential flotation using KBr is time consuming, tedious, and the long preparation time may lead to degradation of the lipoproteins, which are very sensitive to oxidative damage. In addition, with all KBr techniques it is usually necessary to remove the salt by dialysis (often adding a further 12 h to the procedure) before subsequent analytical techniques (e.g. agarose gel electrophoresis) or further processing can be carried out. Moreover, the use of high salt concentrations may cause the removal of surface apolipoproteins from lipoproteins. Self-generated gradients iodixanol in vertical or near-vertical rotors (3–12 ml tubes) considerably simplify the separation procedure. Chylomicron-free plasma is adjusted to a suitable starting density by addition of a small volume of OptiPrep™; overlayered with a small volume of saline, loaded into a centrifuge tube and centrifuged for 2–3 h

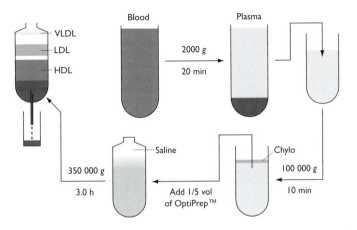

Figure 8.7

Strategy for purifying human plasma lipoproteins in a self-generated iodixanol gradient. VLDL, very low-density lipoproteins; LDL, low-density lipoproteins; HDL, high-density lipoproteins; Chylo, chylomicrons. For more experimental information see Protocol 8.11.

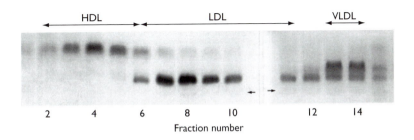

Figure 8.8

Analysis of plasma lipoproteins from iodixanol gradient fractions by agarose gel electrophoresis. Plasma containing 12.5 % (w/v) iodixanol was centrifuged at 353 000 g for 2.5 h in a Beckman NVT100 near-vertical rotor and the gradient unloaded dense end first. Gradient fractions were analyzed by Sudan-black stained agarose gel electrophoresis. HDL, high-density lipoproteins; LDL, low-density lipoproteins; VLDL, very low-density lipoproteins.

(Graham *et al.*, 1996). During the centrifugation, a self-generated gradient forms and the different lipoproteins move to their banding positions; the gradient is collected by tube puncture. The method is summarized in a flow-chart (*Figure 8.7*) and a specimen separation shown in *Figure 8.8*. Not surprisingly the use of isoosmotic (high water activity) iodixanol gradients (compared to those of KBr) reduces the density of the protein-rich HDL much more significantly than LDL and has essentially no effect on the lipid-rich VLDL (*Table 8.5*). The strategy is described in *Protocol 8.11*.

References

Basi, N.S. and Rebois, R.V. (1997) Rate zonal sedimentation of proteins in one hour or less. *Anal. Biochem.* **251:** 103–109.

Bommer, U.A., Burkhardt, N., Jönemann, R., Spahn, C.M.T., Triana-Olonso, F.J. and Nierhaus, K.H. (1997) Ribosomes and polysomes. In: *Subcellular Fractionation – A Practical Approach* (eds J.M. Graham and D. Rickwood). IRL Press at Oxford University Press, Oxford, pp. 271–301.

Chung, B.H., Segrest, J.P., Ray, M.J., Brunzell, J.D., Hokanson, J.E., Krauss, R.M., Beaudrie, K. and Cone, J.T. (1986) Single vertical spin density gradient ultra-centrifugation. *Meth. Enzymol.* **128:** 181–209.

Dettenhoffer, M. and Yu, X-F. (1999) Highly purified human immunodeficiency virus type 1 reveals a virtual absence of Vif in virions *J. Virol.* **73:** 1460–1467.

Eason, R. (1984) Analytical centrifugation. In: *Centrifugation – A Practical Approach* (ed. D. Rickwood). IRL Press at Oxford University Press, Oxford, pp. 251–286.

Ford, T. and Rickwood, D. (1983) Analysis of macromolecules and macromolecular interactions using isopycnic centrifugation. In: *Iodinated Density Gradient Media – A Practical Approach* (ed. D. Rickwood). IRL Press at Oxford University Press, Oxford, pp. 23–42.

Graham, J.M., Higgins, J.A., Gillott, T., Taylor, T., Wilkinson, J., Ford, T. and Billington, D. (1996) A novel method for the rapid separation of plasma lipoproteins using self-generated gradients of iodixanol. *Atherosclerosis* **124:** 125–135.

Gugerli, P. (1984) Isopycnic centrifugation of plant viruses in Nycodenz® density gradients. *J. Virol. Meth.* **9:** 249–258.

Hermens, W.J.M.C., Ter Brake, O., Dijkhuizen, P.A., Sonnemans, M.A.F., Grimm, D., Kleinschmidt, A. and Verhaggen, J. (1999) Purification of recombinant adeno-associated virus by iodixanol gradient ultracentrifugation allows rapid and reproducible preparation of vector stocks for gene transfer in the nervous system. *Human Gene Therapy* **10:** 1885–1891.

Houssais, J.F. (1983) Fractionation of ribonucleoproteins from eukaryotes and prokaryotes. In: *Iodinated Density Gradient Media – A Practical Approach* (ed. D. Rickwood). IRL Press at Oxford University Press, Oxford, pp. 43–67.

Mackness, M. and Durrington, P.N. (1992) Lipoprotein separation and analysis for clinical studies. In: *Lipoprotein Analysis – A Practical Approach* (ed. C.A. Converse and E.R. Skinner). IRL Press at Oxford University Press, Oxford, pp. 1–42.

Møller-Larsen, A. and Christensen, T. (1998) Isolation of a retrovirus from multiple sclerosis patients in self-generated iodixanol gradients *J. Virol. Meth.* **73:** 151–161.

Rickwood, D. (1992) Centrifugal methods for characterizing macromolecules and their interactions. In: *Preparative Centrifugation – A Practical Approach* (ed. D. Rickwood). IRL Press at Oxford University Press, Oxford, pp. 143–186.

Rickwood, D. and Chambers, J.A.A. (1984) Centrifugal methods for characterizing macromolecules and their interactions. In: *Centrifugation – A Practical Approach* (ed. D. Rickwood). IRL Press at Oxford University Press, Oxford, pp. 95–125.

Rickwood, D. and Patel, N.V. (1996) An improved method for the isolation of plasmid DNA using OptiPrep-DAPI gradients. *Mol. Biol. Cell* **7:** 162a.

Steensgard, J., Humphries, S. and Spragg, S.P. (1992) Measurement of sedimentation coefficients. In: *Preparative Centrifugation – A Practical Approach* (ed. D. Rickwood). IRL Press at Oxford University Press, Oxford, pp. 187–232.

Young, B.D. (1984) Measurement of sedimentation coefficients and computer simulation of rate-zonal separations. In: *Centrifugation – A Practical Approach* (ed. D. Rickwood). IRL Press at Oxford University Press, Oxford, pp. 127–159.

Vanden Berghe, D.A. (1983) Comparison of various density-gradient media for the isolation and characterization of animal viruses. In: *Iodinated Density Gradient Media – A Practical Approach* (ed. D. Rickwood). IRL Press at Oxford University Press, Oxford, pp. 175–193.

Zolotukhin, S., Byrne, B.J., Mason, E., Zolotukhin, I., Potter, M., Chesnut, K., Summerford, C., Samulski, R.J. and Muzyczka, N. (1999) Recombinant adeno-associated virus purification using novel methods improves infectious titer and yield. *Gene Therapy* **6**: 973–985.

Protocol 8.1

Purification of plasmid DNA from bacteria using CsCl–EtBr (Rickwood, 1992)

Equipment

Low-speed centrifuge with swinging-bucket rotor to take 200–500 ml bottles

High-speed centrifuge with fixed-angle rotor (8×50 ml tubes)

Ultracentrifuge with Beckman NVT65 (approximately 11 ml tubes) or NVT65.2 (approximately 5 ml tubes) near-vertical rotor

Sealed tubes for the ultracentrifuge rotor

UV illuminator.

Reagents

Lysozyme

Solution A: 50 mM glucose, 10 mM EDTA, 25 mM Tris–HCl, pH 8.0

Solution B: 0.2 M NaOH, 1% (w/v) SDS

Solution C: 3 M sodium acetate (pH 4.8)

TE buffer: 10 mM Tris–HCl (pH 7.4), 2 mM EDTA

Isopropanol

CsCl.

Protocol

This protocol is suitable for 1 l of late log-phase bacteria. Carry out all operations at 0–4°C, except where indicated.

1.   Pellet the bacteria at 2000 g for 20 min.

2.   Wash the bacterial pellet in 100 ml of Solution A and recentrifuge as in step 1.

3.   Resuspend the pellet in 20 ml of Solution A, making sure that the suspension is homogenous.

4.   Add lysozyme to a final concentration of 2 mg ml^{-1}.

5.   After 10 min add 40 ml of Solution B with a gentle swirling action to complete the lysis.

6.   After 5 min add 30 ml of Solution C and leave for another 20 min to precipitate the proteins and some contaminating nucleic acids.

7. Remove the precipitate by centrifugation at 10 000 g for 15 min (fixed-angle rotor).

8. Carefully decant the supernatant and add 55 ml of isopropanol to precipitate the plasmid DNA at −20°C for 20 min.

9. Harvest the crude plasmid DNA by centrifugation at 15 000 g for 5 min.

10. Remove most of the residual isopropanol under vacuum.

11. Dissolve the crude plasmid completely in 18 ml of sterile TE buffer and add 0.65 ml of the ethidium bromide solution.

12. Dissolve completely 1 g of CsCl per ml of solution; the refractive index should be 1.3890.

13. Transfer to tubes for a Beckman NVT65 or NVT65.2 rotor and centrifuge at 350 000 g for 6 h.

14. Visualize the bands under UV light (300 nm).

15. Harvest the lower plasmid DNA containing band (in the middle of the gradient) using a syringe.

Protocol 8.2

Purification of plasmid DNA using DAPI-iodixanol gradients (Rickwood and Patel, 1996)

Equipment

Low-speed centrifuge with swinging-bucket rotor to take 200–500 ml bottles

High-speed centrifuge with fixed-angle rotor (8 × 50 ml tubes)

Ultracentrifuge with near-vertical rotor or low-angle fixed angle rotor (5 ml tube)

Sealed tubes for the ultracentrifuge rotor

UV illuminator.

Reagents

Lysozyme

Solution A: 50 mM glucose, 10 mM EDTA, 25 mM Tris–HCl, pH 8.0

Solution B: 0.2 M NaOH, 1% (w/v) SDS

Solution C: 3 M sodium acetate (pH 4.8)

TE buffer: 10 mM Tris–HCl (pH 7.4), 2 mM EDTA

Isopropanol

70% (v/v) ethanol

OptiPrep™

0.5% (w/v) DAPI.

Protocol

1. Carry out isolation of the crude plasmid DNA using steps 1–10 of *Protocol 8.1*.

2. Wash the pellet in 70% (v/v) ethanol and finally dissolve in 10 ml of TE buffer.

3. To the plasmid solution add OptiPrep™ to a final concentration of 27% (w/v) iodixanol and DAPI to 0.005%.

4. Transfer the solution to a sealed tube for a suitable near-vertical or low-angle fixed angle rotor. With a low-angle fixed-angle rotor (tube size 5 ml) centrifuge at 350 000 g for 12–15 h at 5°C.

5. Observe the result with a UV illuminator and remove the upper plasmid DNA band using a hypodermic syringe.

Protocol 8.3

Sedimentation velocity analysis of proteins in a 5-ml pre-formed sucrose gradient

Equipment

Ultracentrifuge with a swinging-bucket rotor for approximately 5 ml tubes (e.g. Beckman SW50.1)

Two-chamber gradient maker or Gradient Master™

Gradient unloader, tube puncture or automatic aspiration from the top are recommended (see Chapter 4).

Reagents

Protein buffer (PB): 1 mM EDTA, 1 mM dithiothreitol, 2 mM $MgSO_4$ and 0.1% Lubrol PX, 20 mM Hepes–NaOH, pH 8.0. Depending on the protein it may be necessary to include other additives to stabilize the protein such as 100 mM NaCl, chaotropic agents and/or use a different pH, et cetera

Proteins: dissolve the proteins in PB 1–2 mg ml^{-1}

Sucrose solutions: 5% and 20% (w/v) in PB.

Protocol

1. Prepare a 4.8 ml linear 5–20% (w/v) sucrose gradient in tubes for the swinging bucket rotor.

2. Layer 100 µl of protein mixture on top of the gradient and centrifuge at 43 000 r.p.m. for 17 h.

3. Collect the gradient in 0.25-ml fractions using a gradient unloader.

4. Determine the protein distribution by measuring 280 nm absorbance or functional activity.

Note

If the continuous gradient is produced by diffusion of a discontinuous gradient (1.2 ml each of 5, 10, 15 and 20% sucrose) check that the chosen conditions (temperature and time) produce a linear gradient, by measuring the refractive index of blank gradient fractions.

Protocol 8.4

Small-scale sedimentation velocity analysis of proteins in a self-generated iodixanol gradient (Basi and Rebois, 1997)

Equipment

Beckman TLA100, TLA 100.1 or TLA120.1, Sorvall S100-AT3, RP100-AT3, S120-AT3. Larger volume rotors such as the Beckman TLA100.2 or Sorvall S150-AT may be suitable

Gradient unloader, tube puncture or automatic aspiration from the top are recommended (see Chapter 4).

Reagents

OptiPrep™

Diluent: 40 mM Hepes–NaOH, pH 8.0, 2 mM EDTA, 2 mM dithiothreitol, 4 mM MgSO₄ and 0.2% Lubrol PX

Proteins (1.0–2.0 mg ml^{-1}) in 20 mM Hepes–NaOH, pH 8.0, 1 mM EDTA, 1 mM dithiothreitol, 2 mM MgSO₄ and 0.1% Lubrol PX (see *Protocol 8.3* for comments about other suitable media components).

Protocol

1. Mix equal volumes of OptiPrep™ and diluent to produce a 30% (w/v) iodixanol working solution. This can either be used directly as the gradient forming solution or diluted further with solution used to dissolve the proteins as required.

2. Fill a thick-walled open-topped centrifuge to the recommended level with the 30% iodixanol solution.

3. Centrifuge at 350 000 g_{av} for 2–3 h to self-generate the gradient.

4. Allow the rotor to decelerate from 2000 r.p.m. using a controlled deceleration program to allow a smooth reorientation of the gradient.

5. Layer a small volume (10 µl on top of a 0.2 ml gradient; 50 µl on top of a 2.0 ml gradient).

6. Recentrifuge the gradients at approximately 250 000 g_{av} for 1–2 h (depending on tube sedimentation path length). Use controlled programs for acceleration to and deceleration from 2000 r.p.m.

7. Collect the gradient in 0.25 ml fractions using a gradient unloader.

Note

Rotors with 2.0 ml tube sizes may be more practical if the Brandel microfractionator is not available as this is the only unloader that will realistically unload 0.2 ml gradients.

Protocol 8.5

Isolation of polysomes from *E. coli* (Bommer et al., 1997)

Equipment

High-speed centrifuge with 6×250 ml fixed-angle rotor and rotor for microcentrifuge tubes

Ultracentrifuge with swinging-bucket rotor for 14 ml tubes (e.g. Beckman SW41 Ti)

Two-chamber gradient maker or Gradient Master™.

Reagents

Buffer A: 16% (w/v) sucrose, 100 mM NaCl, 6 mM $MgCl_2$, 20 mM Hepes–KOH, pH 7.8

Buffer B: 100 mM NaCl, 6 mM $MgCl_2$, 20 mM Hepes–KOH, pH 7.8

Sucrose solutions: 10% and 40% (w/v) sucrose in 50 mM NH_4Cl, 6 mM $MgCl_2$, 2 mM spermidine, 0.05 mM spermine, 4 mM 2–mercaptoethanol, 20 mM Hepes–KOH, pH 7.5

Lysozyme (50 mg ml^{-1} in water).

Protocol

1. Grow the *E.coli* in 100 ml of a suitable medium (A_{600} = 0.5 units ml^{-1}).

2. Fast cool the cells by pouring the suspension over 100 g of crushed ice in a 250 ml centrifuge tube.

3. Pellet the cells at 2500 g for 5 min.

4. Resuspend the cells in 1 ml of Buffer A and transfer to a 1.5 ml microcentrifuge tube.

5. Add 15 μl of the lysozyme solution and incubate on ice for 2 min.

6. Transfer the cells to −80°C for 1 h.

7. Thaw in an ice-water bath and centrifuge at 32 000 g for 30 min at 2°C.

8. Prepare 13 ml linear 10–40% sucrose gradient in tubes for the ultracentrifuge rotor and bring to 0°C.

9. Dilute the lysate with 3 volumes of Buffer B.

10. Measure the absorbance at A_{260}.

11. Layer the lysate (5–10 A_{260} units/ml) over each gradient and centrifuge at 80 000 g for 7 h at 2°C.

12. Collect the gradient by tube puncture in 0.8 ml fractions.

Protocol 8.6

Isolation of rat liver ribosomal subunits (Bommer *et al.*, 1997)

Equipment

High-speed centrifuge with fixed-angle rotor for 30–50 ml tubes

Ultracentrifuge with fixed-angle rotor (e.g. Beckman 60Ti) and swinging-bucket rotor (e.g. Beckman SW 28)

Potter–Elvehjem homogenizers (5 and 20 ml) with loose-fitting pestles

Two-chamber gradient maker or Gradient Master™

Gradient unloader (tube puncture or upward displacement).

Reagents

Homogenization medium (HM): 0.25 M sucrose, 5 mM $MgCl_2$, 100 mM KCl, 0.2 mM EDTA, 10 mM 2–mercaptoethanol, 50 mM Tris–HCl, pH 7.5

Buffer A: 1.5 mM $MgCl_2$, 50 mM KCl, 10 mM 2-mercaptoethanol, 5 mM Tris–HCl, pH 7.5

Buffer B: 1.5 mM $MgCl_2$, 500 mM KCl, 10 mM 2-mercaptoethanol, 5 mM Tris–HCl, pH 7.5

Puromycin (2.5 mg/ml) in Buffer B

Sodium deoxycholate (10%, w/v) prepared fresh

Sucrose barrier A: 1 M sucrose in 5 mM $MgCl_2$, 100 mM KCl, 10 mM 2-mercaptoethanol, 50 mM Tris–HCl, pH 7.5

Gradient solutions: 5% and 30% (w/v) sucrose in 5 mM $MgCl_2$, 500 mM KCl, 10 mM 2–mercaptoethanol, 5 mM Tris–HCl, pH 7.6 (at 20°C).

Protocol

1. Prepare a rat liver homogenate using five or six strokes of the pestle (500 r.p.m.) of a Potter–Elvehjem homogenizer in HM (2 ml per g of tissue) at 0–4°C.

2. Centrifuge at 12 000 g (0–4°C) for 20 min to remove the nuclei, mitochondria, lysosomes *et cetera*.

3. Collect the upper two-thirds of the supernatant by careful aspiration and filter through four layers of cheesecloth.

4. Add 0.1 volume of the sodium deoxycholate solution and mix gently.

5. Layer over 0.6 volume of sucrose barrier A in the ultracentrifuge fixed-angle rotor and centrifuge at 130 000 g for 12–16 h.

6. Remove the supernatant and rinse the surface of the ribosomal pellet with Buffer A by careful swirling than resuspend crudely in this buffer using a glass rod.

7. Complete the resuspension using a small Potter–Elvehjem homogenizer (approximately 20 mg ml^{-1}). This is equivalent to an A_{260} units ml^{-1} of 260.

8. Adjust the KCl concentration to 500 mM and add the puromycin solution (1 mg per 100 mg of ribosomes).

9. Add Buffer B to adjust the suspension to 10 mg ribosomes ml^{-1} and incubate on ice for 30 min and at 37°C for 15 min.

10. Centrifuge at 10 000 g for 5 min to remove any debris.

11. Prepare linear gradients of 15–30% sucrose in tubes for the SW28 rotor (36 ml).

12. Layer 3 ml of the dissociated ribosomes over the gradient and centrifuge at 30 000 g for 14 h at 20°C.

13. Collect the gradient by tube puncture or upward displacement and monitor the effluent at A_{260} to identify the two peaks of 40-S and 60-S subunits.

Note

The purity of the subunits can be further enhanced by further centrifugation procedures, for information on this and other ribonucleoprotein methods, see Bommer *et al.* (1997).

Protocol 8.7

Concentration and purification of Sendai virus (100–200 ml) using a large volume fixed-angle rotor

Equipment

Low-speed centrifuge with swinging-bucket rotor (50–100 ml tubes)

Ultracentrifuge with a fixed-angle rotor accommodating 90–100 ml (e.g. Beckman 45Ti).

Reagents

Sucrose solutions: 35, 45 and 55% (w/w) in buffered saline or culture medium.

Protocol

Carry out all operations at 4°C.

1. Clarify the virus-containing fluid at 3000 g for 20 min.

2. Layer the clarified fluid (approximately 75 ml) over 20 ml of 55% (w/w) sucrose in tubes for the ultracentrifuge rotor and centrifuge at 100 000 g for 90 min.

3. Remove as much as possible of the supernatant from above the virus band at the interface.

4. Harvest the virus in 4–5 ml of the dense sucrose cushion.

5. Dilute the virus suspension with 2 volumes of buffered saline.

6. In new tubes for the same rotor layer 20 ml each of 55, 45 and 35% sucrose and then the virus suspension to fill the tube. If the volume of virus does not fill the tube, layer buffered saline on top.

7. Centrifuge at 150 000 g for 4–6 h.

8. Harvest the banded virus.

9. Dialyze the gradient fractions against buffered saline.

Protocol 8.8

Concentration and purification of rAAV in a discontinuous iodixanol gradient (Zolotukhin *et al.*, 1999)

Equipment

High-speed centrifuge with fixed-angle rotor

Fixed-angle rotor with approximately 39 ml sealed tubes capable of approximately 350 000g (e.g. Beckman 70Ti or Sorvall T865).

Reagents

10×Phosphate-buffered saline containing 10 mM $MgCl_2$ and 25 mM KCl (10×PBS-MK)

PBS-MK: PBS containing 1 mM $MgCl_2$ and 2.5 mM KCl

2 M NaCl in PBS-MK

OptiPrep™

Working solution (WS): 54% (w/v) iodixanol: mix 9 volumes of OptiPrep with 1 volume 10×PBS-MK

Gradient solutions:

15% (w/v) iodixanol: 1.5 volumes of WS + 2.7 vol of 2 M NaCl + 1.2 volumes of PBS-MK

25% (w/v) iodixanol: 2.5 volumes of WS + 2.9 volumes of PBS-MK

40% (w/v) iodixanol: 4.0 volumes of WS + 1.5 volumes of PBS-MK

Protocol

Carry out all operations at 4°C.

1. Clarify the cell lysate by centrifugation at 4000 g for 20 min.

2. Underlayer 10–15 ml of clarified lysate with 9 ml of 15% iodixanol; 6 ml of 25% iodixanol, 5 ml of 40% iodixanol and 5 ml of the 54% iodixanol working solution.

3. Centrifuge at 350 000 g_{av} for 1 h at 18°C. Use a slow acceleration and deceleration program (up to and below 2000 r.p.m.), or turn off the brake below 2000 r.p.m. during deceleration.

4. Either collect the whole gradient in 1–2 ml fractions dense end first (e.g. tube puncture) or use a syringe inserted at the 40%/60% interface to aspirate 4 ml of the 40% layer which contains the rAAV.

Note

The 1 M NaCl in the 15% iodixanol minimizes the tendency for soluble proteins to adhere to the virus.

Protocol 8.9

Concentration and purification of virus using a self-generated iodixanol gradient

Equipment

Low-speed centrifuge with swinging-bucket rotor (50–100 ml tubes)

Ultracentrifuge with any fixed-angle rotor (with approximately 40 ml tubes) that is used routinely to pellet the virus. For gradient purification: any vertical, near-vertical rotor with tube capacity of approximately 12 ml and capable of approximately 350 000 g.

Reagents

OptiPrep™

Diluent: 0.85% (w/v) NaCl, 60 mM Hepes–NaOH, pH 7.4

WS of 50% (w/v) iodixanol: mix 5 volumes of OptiPrep™ and 1 volume of diluent

Hepes buffered saline (HBS): 0.85% NaCl (w/v), 10 mM Hepes–NaOH, pH 7.4.

Protocol

Carry out all operations at 4°C.

1.   Clarify the virus suspension by centrifugation at 1000 g for 10 min.

2.   Transfer a known volume of the supernatant to tubes for the fixed-angle rotor and underlay with a cushion of 5 ml of WS.

3.   Centrifuge at 50 000–100 000 g for 1–2 h (depending on the virus) to band the virus sharply at the WS interface. Allow the rotor to decelerate from 1000 r.p.m. without the brake.

4.   Remove all of the supernatant except for a volume equal to the volume of cushion.

5.   Mix the residual contents of the tubes. This will produce a concentrated virus suspension in 25% (w/v) iodixanol.

6.   Transfer the suspension to sealed tubes for a vertical, near-vertical rotor.

7.   Any tubes that are not filled should be topped up and mixed with 25% iodixanol.

8.   Centrifuge at 350 000 g_{av} for 2.4 h and use either a controlled deceleration program or turn off the brake below 2000 r.p.m.

9.   Either harvest the virus band or unload the entire gradient by tube puncture, or other suitable method. The Herpes virus will band in the lower third of the tube.

Note

This method was developed for Herpes Virus. For other viruses, it may be necessary to modulate the iodixanol concentration used for the self-generated gradient.

Protocol 8.10

Fractionation of lipoproteins by sequential flotation using KBr

This procedure is suitable for approximately 80 ml of plasma and is a useful method for compositional analysis but it can be scaled down as required. Fixed-angle rotors of a low angle should be used to reduce the distance traveled by the lipoproteins.

Equipment

High speed centrifuge with fixed-angle rotor (8×50 ml)

Ultracentrifuge with fixed-angle rotor to accommodate approximately 38 ml tubes (e.g. Beckman 60Ti)

Refractometer.

Reagents

High-density salt solution: 153 g of NaCl, 354 g of KBr, 100 µg EDTA in 1 l of water. The density of this solution should be 1.33 g ml^{-1}, check this periodically using a refractometer.

Protocol

1. Divide the plasma between two tubes for the high-speed fixed angle rotor and centrifuge at approximately 50 000 g for 30 min to float any chylomicrons.

2. Remove the infranatant beneath the milky layer of chylomicrons.

3. Transfer the chylomicron-free plasma to tubes for the ultracentrifuge rotor and centrifuge at 100 000 g for 20 h at 10–15°C.

4. Remove the floating layer of VLDL together with 1–2 ml of the immediate infranatant.

5. Resuspend the pellet, which contains plasma proteins, LDL and HDL in the remaining infranatant and measure this volume.

6. Mix this solution with the dense salt solution to give a density of 1.063 g ml^{-1} using the equation in Chapter 3.

7. Centrifuge at 100 000 g for 28 h at 10–15°C.

8. Remove the floating layer of LDL and again resuspend the pellet in the residual infranatant and adjust the density of this to 1.21 g ml^{-1} by further addition of the dense salt solution using the equation in Chapter 3.

9. Centrifuge at 100 000 g for 48 h at 10–15°C.

10. Remove the floating layer of HDL.

11. Dialyze the LDL and HDL fractions to reduce the high salt concentration.

Protocol 8.11

Fractionation of lipoproteins in self-generated gradients of iodixanol (Graham *et al.*, 1996)

This procedure is suitable for approximately 2–10 ml of plasma, although it can be scaled up by using additional tubes. It is a useful method for both density analysis of lipoproteins and also for small-scale preparation of lipoproteins for compositional analysis.

Equipment

Any vertical or near-vertical rotor (sedimentation path-length of approximately 17 mm or less) for an ultra- or microultracentrifuge. Tube volumes of 2–12 ml are normally suitable, e.g. Beckman TLN100 (3.1-ml tubes), NVT65.2 (5-ml tubes) and VTi65.1 (11-ml tubes)

Optiseal™ tubes are the recommended tubes for Beckman vertical and near-vertical rotors.

Ultracentrifuge fixed-angle rotor (e.g. TLA100.4) or high speed centrifuge with fixed-angle rotor (8×15 ml).

Reagents

OptiPrep™

HBS: 0.85% (w/v) NaCl, 10 mM Hepes–NaOH, pH 7.4.

Protocol

1. Remove chylomicrons from the plasma by centrifugation at 100 000 g for 10 min in the TLA100.4 or for larger volumes use the high speed centrifuge fixed-angle rotor at 50 000 g for 30 min.

2. Mix 4 volumes of plasma with 1 volume of OptiPrep™ (12% iodixanol final concentration) and transfer to a suitable OptiSeal™ tube (approx 90% of tube volume).

3. Layer Solution B on top to fill the tube. With a vertical rotor, first underlayer with 0.2–0.5 ml of 20% iodixanol; this prevents dense particles reaching the wall of the tube.

4. After sealing the tube, centrifuge at approximately 350 000 g_{av} for 2.5–3 h, using slow acceleration to and deceleration from 2000 r.p.m.

5. Collect the gradient in 0.1–0.2 ml fractions by tube puncture and analyze the fractions directly as required.

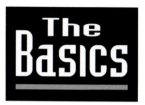

List of manufacturers and technical support sources

There are so many varieties of bench-top and floor-standing low-speed, bench-top high-speed centrifuges and microfuges commercially available, that a list of manufacturers and suppliers would cover many pages if it attempted to be comprehensive. Moreover, many of these are available from general scientific supplies companies and will be known to the administrative sections of academic and commercial laboratories. Instead, this list is restricted to the provision of full contact details of the major producers of ultracentrifuge and floor-standing high-speed centrifuges, of the specialty equipment used for making and collecting density gradients and of density gradient media.

Where manufacturers have world-wide organizations contact details are provided only for the USA and UK.

Major manufacturers of ultracentrifuges and floor-standing high-speed centrifuges

There are essentially three brand names of these machines: Beckman, Sorvall and Hitachi. In North America and Europe, Hitachi machines are supplied by Kendro Laboratory Products (see below).

Beckman centrifuges

In the USA: Beckman Coulter Inc., 4300 North Harbor Boulevard, PO Box 3100, Fullerton, CA 92834-3100, USA. Tel: +1 714 871 4848. Fax: +1 714 773 8283.

In the UK: Beckman Coulter (UK) Ltd., Oakley Court, Kingsmead Business Park, London Road, High Wycombe, Bucks HP11 1JG, UK. Tel: +44 (0)1494441 181. Fax: +44 (0)1494 447558. E-mail: beckmancoulter_uk@beckman. com. Website: www.beckman-coulter.com.

Sorvall and Hitachi centrifuges

In the USA: Kendro Laboratory Products, 31, Pecks Lane, Newtown, CT 006470-2337, USA. Tel: 800 522 7746. Fax: +1 205 270 2166. E-mail: info@kendro.com.

In the UK: Kendro Laboratory Products, Stortford Hall Park, Bishop's Stortford, Herts CM23 5GZ, UK. Tel: +44 (0)1279 827700. Fax: +44 (0)1279 827750. E-mail: kendro@kendro. co.uk.

Website: www.sorvall.com.

Gradient makers and unloaders

Auto Densiflow Gradient Fractionator

In the USA: Labconco Corp., 8811 Prospect Avenue, Kansas City, MO 64132-2696, USA. Tel: 800 821 5525; +1 816 333 8811. Fax: +1 816 363 0130. E-mail: labconco@labconco.com.

In the UK: Genetic Research Instrumentation Ltd., Gene House, Queensborough Lane, Rayne, Braintree, Essex CM7 8TF, UK. Tel: +44 (0)1376 332900. Fax: +44 (0)1376 344724. E-mail: gri@dial.pipex.com. Website: www.labconco.com.

Axis-Shield Gradient Unloader

See 'Iodinated density gradient media'

Beckman-Coulter Fraction Recovery System

See 'Beckman centrifuges'

Gradient Master and Gradient Mate gradient makers

Biocomp Instruments Inc, 650 Churchill Row, Fredricton, New Brunswick, Canada, E3B 1P6. Tel: 800 561 4221; +1 506 453 4812. E-mail: dhc@unb.ca.

Density gradient media

Colloidal silica gradient media

In the USA: Amersham Pharmacia Biotech, 800 Centennial Avenue, PO box 1327, Piscataway, NJ 08855-1327, USA. Tel: 800 526 3593. Fax: +1 877 295 8102. E-mail: apbcsus@ am.apbiotech.com.

In the UK: Amersham Pharmacia Biotech, Amersham Place, Little Chalfont, Bucks HP7 9NA, UK. Tel: +44 (0)870 606 1921; +44 (0)1494 542179. E-mail: ts-molbio.gb@eu. apbiotech.com.

Website: www.apbiotech.com.

Iodinated density gradient media (Lymphoprep™, Polymorphprep™, Nycoprep™ 1.077, Nycoprep™ 1.068, Nycoprep™ Universal, Nycodenz® and OptiPrep™) and Polysucrose.

Axis-Shield PoC, PO Box 6863, Rodeløkka, N0504 Oslo, Norway. Tel: +47 22 04 20 26. Fax: +47 22 04 20 01. E-mail: bjh@no.axis-shield.com. Website: www.axis-shield-poc.com/ density.

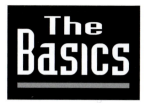

Index